Psychotherapeutic Support for Family Caregivers of People With Dementia

About the Author

Gabiele Wilz, PhD, is Head of the Department of Counseling and Clinical Intervention and Director of the Psychotherapeutic Outpatient Clinic and CBT qualification at the Friedrich Schiller University Jena since 2009. She studied psychology in Marburg, received her PhD in 1998 at University of Leipzig, and worked from 1998 to 2003 as Assistant Professor at the University of Leipzig in the Department of Medical Psychology and Medical Sociology. From 2003 to 2008 she was Professor of Clinical and Health Psychology at the Technical University of Berlin. She is a licensed clinical psychologist and clinical supervisor with licensure in cognitive-behavioral psychotherapy.

Psychotherapeutic Support for Family Caregivers of People With Dementia

The Tele.TAnDem Manual

Gabriele Wilz
Marlena L. Itz (Translator)

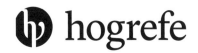

Library of Congress Cataloging in Publication information for the print version of this book is available via the Library of Congress Marc Database under the LC Control Number 2023945513

Library and Archives Canada Cataloguing in Publication
Title: Psychotherapeutic support for family caregivers of people with dementia : the Tele.TAnDem manual / Gabriele Wilz ; Marlena L. Itz (translator).
Other titles: Therapeutische Unterstützung für pflegende Angehörige von Menschen mit Demenz. English
Names: Wilz, Gabriele, 1966- author.
Description: The present volume is a translation of Therapeutische Unterstützung für pflegende Angehörige von Menschen mit Demenz. Das Tele. TAnDem Behandlungsprogramm by Gabriele Wilz, Denise Schinköthe, & Tanja Kalytta Copyright © 2015 by Hogrefe Verlag GmbH & Co. KG. -- Title page verso. | Includes bibliographical references.
Identifiers: Canadiana (print) 20230526551 | Canadiana (ebook) 20230526594 | ISBN 9780889376311 (softcover) | ISBN 9781616766313 (PDF) | ISBN 9781613346310 (EPUB)
Subjects: LCSH: Cognitive therapy—Handbooks, manuals, etc. | LCSH: Caregivers—Psychology—Handbooks, manuals, etc. | LCSH: Dementia—Patients—Care—Handbooks, manuals, etc.
Classification: LCC RC489.C63 W5513 2024 | DDC 616.89/1425—dc23

Original title: *Therapeutische Unterstützung für pflegende Angehörige von Menschen mit Demenz. Das Tele.TAnDem Behandlungsprogramm* by Gabriele Wilz, Denise Schinköthe, & Tanja Kalytta
© 2015 by Hogrefe Verlag GmbH & Co. KG
Translated by Marlena L. Itz

© 2024 by Hogrefe Publishing
www.hogrefe.com

The authors and publisher have made every effort to ensure that the information contained in this text is in accord with the current state of scientific knowledge, recommendations, and practice at the time of publication. In spite of this diligence, errors cannot be completely excluded. Also, due to changing regulations and continuing research, information may become outdated at any point. The authors and publisher disclaim any responsibility for any consequences which may follow from the use of information presented in this book.

Registered trademarks are not noted specifically as such in this publication. The use of descriptive names, registered names, and trademarks does not imply, even in the absence of a specific statement, that such names are exempt from the relevant protective laws and regulations and therefore free for general use.

The cover image is an agency photo depicting models. Use of the photo on this publication does not imply any connection between the content of this publication and any person depicted in the cover image.
Cover image: © TatyanaGI - iStock.com
Author photo, back cover: © Anne Günther - University of Jena, Germany

PUBLISHING OFFICES
USA: Hogrefe Publishing Corporation, 44 Merrimac St., Suite 207, Newburyport, MA 01950
Phone 978 255 3700; E-mail customersupport@hogrefe.com
EUROPE: Hogrefe Publishing GmbH, Merkelstr. 3, 37085 Göttingen, Germany
Phone +49 551 99950 0, Fax +49 551 99950 111; E-mail publishing@hogrefe.com

SALES & DISTRIBUTION
USA: Hogrefe Publishing, Customer Services Department,
30 Amberwood Parkway, Ashland, OH 44805
Phone 800 228 3749, Fax 419 281 6883; E-mail customersupport@hogrefe.com
UK: Hogrefe Publishing, c/o Marston Book Services Ltd., 160 Eastern Ave., Milton Park, Abingdon, OX14 4SB
Phone +44 1235 465577, Fax +44 1235 465556; E-mail direct.orders@marston.co.uk
EUROPE: Hogrefe Publishing, Merkelstr. 3, 37085 Göttingen, Germany
Phone +49 551 99950 0, Fax +49 551 99950 111; E-mail publishing@hogrefe.com

OTHER OFFICES
CANADA: Hogrefe Publishing, 82 Laird Drive, East York, Ontario, M4G 3V1
SWITZERLAND: Hogrefe Publishing, Länggass-Strasse 76, 3012 Bern

No part of this book may be reproduced, stored in a retrieval system or transmitted, in any form or by any means, electronic, mechanical, photocopying, microfilming, recording or otherwise, without written permission from the publisher.

Printed and bound in Germany

ISBN 978-0-88937-631-1 (print) • ISBN 978-1-61676-631-3 (PDF) • ISBN 978-1-61334-631-0 (EPUB)
https://doi.org/10.1027/00631-000

Contents

Foreword		1
Preface		3
1	**Demands, Burden, and Health Impact of Caregiving**	**5**
1.1	Introduction	5
1.2	Overview of Specific Caregiver Burden in Dementia	5
1.3	Models and Predictors for Burden and Coping With Caregiving	7
1.4	Family Caregivers' Coping Strategies	9
1.5	Positive Aspects of Caregiving	9
2	**Need for and Effectiveness of Psychosocial Interventions**	**11**
2.1	Need for Helpful Family Caregiver Interventions	11
2.2	Demands for Helpful Family Caregiver Interventions	12
2.3	CBT-Based Caregiver Interventions: Content, Evaluation, and Recommendations	12
2.4	Concept and Evaluation of the Tele.TAnDem Intervention	15
3	**Helpful Information on Dementia and Caregiving-Specific Issues for Family Caregivers**	**19**
3.1	Illness-Specific Topics	19
3.2	Medical Questions	22
3.3	Care-Related Questions	22
3.4	Legal Questions	23
3.5	Financial Questions	23
4	**Diagnostic Tools for Caregiving of People With Dementia**	**25**
4.1	Questionnaires for Family Caregivers	25
4.2	Questionnaires for the Subjective Assessment of Behavioral Problems in Dementia Patients	27
4.3	Assessment of the Severity of Dementia	27
5	**Therapist Attitude and Relationship Building**	**29**
5.1	The Caregivers Are Caregiving Experts	30
5.2	Normalizing and Depathologizing Counseling	30
5.3	Family Caregivers Are Doing Their Best: Appreciation and Validation of Their Efforts	30
5.4	Isolation and Severe Suffering: Empathy and Patience	32
5.5	Unchangeable Burdens and Loss of Control: Confrontation and Acceptance	33

6	**Therapy Topics, Intervention Methods, and Framework**	**35**
6.1	Individualized Therapy	35
6.2	Setting	36
6.3	Therapy Process and Structure of the Sessions	36
6.4	Work Between Sessions: Therapeutic Homework	37
7	**First Session and Relationship Building**	**39**
7.1	Goals of the Module	39
7.2	Therapeutic Approach	39
8	**"I Grew Up in the Countryside, and That Was a Given There": Changing Dysfunctional Thoughts and Appraisals**	**47**
8.1	Goals of the Module	48
8.2	Therapeutic Approach	48
9	**"You Are Still at Home Here!" – Dealing With Challenging Behavior**	**59**
9.1	Goals of the Module	59
9.2	Therapeutic Approach	61
10	**"Anger Is Completely Normal" – Stress Management and Emotion Regulation**	**77**
10.1	Goals of the Module	77
10.2	Therapeutic Approach	78
11	**"And What About Me?" – Self-Care and Value-Based Activities**	**87**
11.1	Goals of the Module	87
11.2	Therapeutic Approach	88
12	**"From the Diagnosis Until Death" – Dealing With Change, Loss, and Grief**	**99**
12.1	Goals of the Module	99
12.2	Therapeutic Approach	100
12.3	The Time After the Death of the Person With Dementia	113
13	**"I Need to Do It on My Own" – Support Options for Family Caregivers of Persons With Dementia**	**117**
13.1	Goals of the Module	117
13.2	Identifying the Need for Assistance	118
13.3	Overcoming Barriers to Utilizing Support	119
13.4	Finding the Right Time for Support	120
13.5	Searching for Support Options	123
13.6	Difficulties Regarding Utilization of Support	125
14	**Nursing-Home Placement – When the Limits of Home Care Have Been Reached**	**131**
14.1	Goals of the Module	131
14.2	Decision-Making Factors	131
14.3	Support in Decision Making	135
14.4	Care in an Emergency	138
14.5	Dealing With the Decision	139
14.6	Therapeutic Procedure for Intolerable Caregiving Situations	142

15	**Completion of Therapy**	**147**
15.1	Goals of the Module	147
15.2	Therapeutic Approach	147

References **151**

Appendix **159**

Foreword

Books for mental health professionals are published every year, sometimes updating what is already known, sometimes rewording what we already know, but rarely providing something very new and important – what we don't know and what is important for us to know. This book by Gabriele Wilz, *Psychotherapeutic Support for Family Caregivers of People With Dementia*, is a welcome, important, indeed much needed and exciting, contribution to the field. And I feel privileged to be able to write its Foreword.

As any practicing therapist knows, people rarely change by simply telling them to do something different. Yet, the extent to which therapists intervene when working clinically with a caregiver – and I must confess that I am guilty of this myself – is telling them "It is important to take care of yourself." What is needed beyond this simple behavioral suggestion is how to deal with the emotions – guilt, stress, apprehension, resentment, depression, anger – that might make it difficult for them to care for themselves. What therapists need is to help the caregiver learn, sometimes painstakingly so, how to develop a new and very difficult caregiver script, one that involves significant changes in their emotions, thinking, and behavior. This volume provides clinicians with clinical guidelines for helping caregivers adopt this new, complicated, and emotionally difficult script.

This volume describes how therapists can work clinically with patients or clients who are caring for a significant other who is suffering from dementia. Among the many difficulties associated with dementia are short-term memory loss, language problems, orientation difficulties, difficulty in caring for themselves, and impaired cognitive functioning. Depending on the severity of impairment, cognitively impaired individuals typically require the assistance of others to get through the day. Currently, it is estimated that over 50 million people in the world suffer from some form of dementia – most typically Alzheimer's disease. Moreover, this alarming statistic is likely to increase as individuals live longer.

Although medical research has been focusing on ways to better understand dementia, it has yet to come up with a cure or even an effective treatment. Knowledge of the psychological aspects of dementia similarly leave much to be desired, and we are limited in our understanding of what therapists need to know and do to help caregivers cope with the task of helping loved ones. In short, there is a crying need for clinical guidelines to help therapists in working with caregivers, and this volume fills this much-needed void.

Caring for a cognitively impaired significant other is probably one of the most difficult experiences one is likely to encounter in one's lifetime. I say this not only from my work as a therapist, but also from personal experience. It is a totally new world, whereby the rules for day-to-day interactions with a loved one are likely to be different from anything one has experienced in the past. It can be unbelievably challenging emotionally, cognitively, and behaviorally. Caregivers are likely to experience a myriad of emotions, such as stress, anger, guilt, depression, exasperation – just to mention a few. Cognitively, there is confusion – being at a loss in trying to understand what is happening to one's significant other along with confusion about what to do in day-to-day interactions. Behaviorally, a caregiver's own life is disrupted, and they find themselves having difficulty personally functioning as they had in the past. Without clinical guidelines for working with caregivers, therapists are likely to end up having their own emotional, cognitive, and behavioral difficulties professionally.

Psychotherapeutic Support for Family Caregivers of People With Dementia offers highly sophisticated clinical guidelines, describing everything a therapist needs to know in working with caregivers. It describes not only what to do and why to do it, but also the behavioral, cognitive, and emotional obstacles that can undermine therapeutic progress. Moreover, it contains several modules that can allow the practicing clinician to personalize the intervention to the specific needs of the patient.

In short, this is an invaluable volume that provides practicing therapists with clinically relevant and empirically grounded therapeutic guidelines for working with the ever-increasing number of caregivers who are confronted with the challenging task of caring for a loved one. In addition to offering helpful information about dementia, it also describes the burden put on caregivers and validates the very important role of support in their lives. The therapy modules that can be tailored to the needs of the patient include guidelines on how to solve the numerous situational challenges one is likely to encounter in caring for a loved one; strategies for dealing with the wide range of emotions associated with caregiving; and ways to achieve the all-important goal of accepting those aspects of one's life circumstances that cannot be changed. Not only is this clinically meaningful, but research evidence exists that it indeed makes a significant positive impact on the psychological and physical well-being of caregivers.

Marvin R. Goldfried, PhD
Stony Brook University
New York, USA

Preface

The majority of caregiving responsibilities for older people is shouldered by family members. Due to the increasing number of people with dementia worldwide and the amount of care and assistance they require, supporting caregivers is becoming an increasingly important issue in health care. Without family members who take on most of the care in private households, it would not be possible to ensure sufficient assistance for people with dementia, as well as for older family members who need help in general.

Although family caregivers are usually healthy, they are at great risk of developing mental and physical health problems such as depressive and anxiety symptoms, insomnia, and exhaustion.

This raises the question of why the enormously helpful strategies of psychotherapy are usually not provided for the heavily burdened caring relatives, to prevent mental illness and physical impairments. Up to now, cognitive-behavioral therapy (CBT) for family caregivers has been hardly addressed in the training of psychotherapists, even though some research studies have evaluated comprehensive psychotherapeutic concepts in this area. Moreover, as a significant preventive intervention, CBT for family caregivers is not regularly established in health care systems.

Because of this need, I have continuously pursued the goal of developing and evaluating specific psychotherapeutically sound support concepts for family caregivers. As a result, the Tele.TAnDem concept was created, which was published in 2015 in cooperation with Dr. Denise Schinköthe and Tanja Kalytta from my research group (Wilz, G., Schinköthe, D., & Kalytta, T. (2015). Therapeutische Unterstützung für pflegende Angehörige von Menschen mit Demenz. Das Tele.TAnDem-Behandlungsprogramm. Göttingen: Hogrefe (Psychotherapeutic support for family caregivers of people with dementia. The Tele.TAnDem concept).

Dr. Marlena L. Itz has translated the English version of the handbook in an intensive, careful, and outstanding manner. On basis of this translation, all parts of the text were considered in a joint exchange and linguistic revisions were discussed. Furthermore, I have undertaken relevant updates and have adapted the topics with regard to international requirements.

The handbook is based on cognitive behavioral therapy. In 10 different modules main typical caregiving topics and useful intervention strategies such as cognitive restructuring, emotion regulation, problem solving, self-care, and coping with loss and grief are addressed. Furthermore, specific aspects of acceptance and commitment therapy are integrated, because many aspects of the disease and the caregiving situation cannot be changed. Helping caregivers to manage and accept the negative emotions and cognitions accompanying such a difficult experience (e.g. anger, grief, shame, guilt, anxiety, and depression) is another central objective of the intervention.

The book aims to provide comprehensive and specific guidance as how to work psychotherapeutically with family caregivers. This goal is realized through clear instructions, case examples, work sheets, exercises, and precise explanations. Special features of the book are the comprehensive dialogues of real therapy sessions and a focus on how to build and maintain a helpful therapeutic alliance and motivation to change for family caregivers. The intervention is suitable for various settings such as group, face-to-face, or remote therapy forms (telephone and online/web-based therapy). In several RCTs and qualitative studies, the therapy concept has been positively evaluated.

So far, the caregivers evaluated this specific psychotherapeutic support as particular helpful, as the following quotations illustrate:

> "Discussing and analyzing stressful situations when I got out of my skin at the end of my nerves and yelled at my innocent, ill husband. Working together on how to cope with these feelings, without affecting my husband. How I let off steam, was very helpful."

> "I have gained a much better understanding of the disease and can react more calmly to the problems."

> "By listening, responding to me, being taken seriously and noticed, problem solutions were worked out, emotions were captured and taken seriously, to develop other perspectives on situations helped me and strengthening my person."

"Through the consultation, I have learned to take more care of myself and to do something for myself. I try not to lose sight of that. The word mindfulness has taken on a very special meaning for me!"

"I try hard to get space for myself. The realization that I can't give up completely if I want to persevere, that this is even essential."

"It was a blessing that I participated in this therapy and the only effective help. I am infinitely grateful for that!"

"The psychological support was perfect! Please don't change anything!"

I am very happy that a translation of the manual is now available. I hope it will be helpful for therapists and other professionals, as well as for family caregivers.

Jena, in February 2023   Gabriele Wilz

1 Demands, Burden, and Health Impact of Caregiving

This chapter provides an overview of the specific burden caregivers may experience while providing care for a family member living with dementia. Models and predictors that may play a crucial role in the individual experience of burden are presented as well as coping strategies and positive aspects of providing care.

1.1 Introduction

There are currently 57.4 million people worldwide living with dementia, which is predicted to triple by the year 2050 (GBD 2019 Dementia Forecasting Collaborators, 2022). As there is presently no causal treatment for dementia, ensuring the care of people with dementia will become a challenge in the coming decades for health policy makers and families. Contrary to the stereotype of "nursing-home placement," around 69% of people suffering from dementia are cared for at home, with almost two thirds of them cared for exclusively by family members, mainly wives, daughters, or daughters-in-law (Wimo et al., 2018).

Due to the specific symptoms of dementia, family members are confronted with particularly burdensome problem situations that can constantly change daily and as the disease progresses. Caring for someone with dementia can thus be described as an extremely demanding task. The caregiver must constantly overcome new challenges in daily life and in relation to the changes in the person with dementia. This large number of stressors often causes health-related impairments. In addition to the increased health impairments (Cheng, 2017) and mortality rates (Schulz & Beach, 1999), caregivers of people with dementia have considerably more severe impairments in mental and physical health compared to comparable healthy populations or caregivers of other chronically ill care recipients (Pinquart & Sörensen, 2003).

In particular, 30–60% of caregivers have reported clinically meaningful depressive symptoms (Barrera-Caballero et al., 2021; Collins & Kishita, 2020; Joling et al., 2015), higher prevalence rates of anxiety (32%, Kaddour & Kishita, 2020), and higher rates of comorbidity of both depression and anxiety (32–54%, Barrera-Caballero et al., 2021; Joling et al., 2015) and lower quality of life (Karg et al., 2018). Health impairments have also been shown for physiological parameters such as higher blood pressure, risk of cardiovascular diseases, reduced immune function, and a longer healing time for wounds (Gouin et al., 2008; Mausbach et al., 2007; von Känel et al., 2008). Particularly, female caregivers, who make up more than 70% of all caregivers, are especially burdened (Barrera-Caballero et al., 2021; Joling et al., 2015; Kaddour & Kishita, 2020). Accordingly, Collins and Kishita (2020) reported 1.45 times higher odds of women having depression compared to male caregivers.

Additionally, when caregivers receive insufficient support, their experience of burden is particularly pronounced (Holst & Edberg, 2011). Thus, due to the above-mentioned health consequences for the caregivers on the one hand, as well as the increasing numbers of dementia cases due to demographic changes, on the other hand, there is an urgent need to preserve at-home care and support caregivers in this challenging task.

1.2 Overview of Specific Caregiver Burden in Dementia

When caring for a family member with dementia, caregivers face an abundance of complex, challenging, and time-consuming demands. Experiences and results from our studies provide evidence of the long-lasting burden of being involved in caregiving, which lasted an average of 5 years. For example, family caregivers reported spending an average of 11 hours per day providing care, with more than half of the participants (52%) reporting that they had to ensure round-the-clock care. For 26% of study participants, this meant that they either could not leave the dementia sufferer alone during the day or only for less than 1 hour. The high need for care was due to attending to orientation disorders, confusion, self-threatening behavior, or personality changes, as well as performing care tasks (household management, assistance with food and fluid intake), helping with personal hygiene, especially for incontinence (64% of the people with dementia), visiting public authorities, doctor visits, and engaging with the person with dementia. At the time of the initial assessment, 40% of the family caregivers provided nighttime care in addition to daytime care: Family caregivers had to help the person with dementia up to 12 times per night, mainly with using the toilet or changing incontinence pads and/or bed linens. These tasks are particularly burdensome for caregivers who care for a physically mobile person with dementia whose nightly disturbances increase (see also Miyamoto et al., 2002).

Moreover, family caregiving often occurs without a prior deliberate decision-making process. It is often seen as a nonquestionable "matter of course." Accordingly, family caregivers are mostly unprepared for the ensuing tasks and burden. Here it is important to note that, due to the changing symptoms, which are in turn dependent on the severity of the disease, caregivers are confronted with various and changing caregiving situations. In the following list, the most important demands regarding guidance, support, and caregiving tasks are summarized:

- Support for the family member with dementia in daily tasks. In the beginning, assistance with complex day-to-day activities is necessary (e.g., shopping, handling of financial matters), which are then fully taken over by the caregiver. As the course of the disease progresses, simpler everyday activities (such as getting dressed, preparation and intake of meals) require more intensive guidance and support from the caregiver.
- Taking care of personal hygiene and assisting with mobility (e.g., walking, going to bed) at advanced stages of the disease.
- Attending to the relative with dementia when temporal, local, and personal disorientation increases.
- Dealing with dementia-related cognitive impairments, neurological symptoms (e.g., speech disorders), gait disorders, incontinence, and other consequences of dementia.
- Dealing with restlessness, anxiety and depression, day-night rhythm disorders, aggressiveness, social withdrawal, and passivity, as well as delusional symptoms.
- Dealing with challenging behavior in private surroundings and in public.
- Stabilizing and promoting remaining abilities and skills as well as mental well-being through meaningful activation and involvement of the relative with dementia in everyday life.

However, caregiving not only places special demands on the organization and arrangement of daily life and requires the appropriation of new skills for the support and care of the impaired person, family caregivers must also adapt mentally in order to perceive and accept the changes in a person close to them, as well as to learn to deal with these changes and integrate them into their relationship. The challenge in dementia caregiving lies, therefore, in coping mentally and emotionally with the disease and processing one's own emotional distress and losses. In particular, the following aspects describe the situation in which family caregivers find themselves.

- Due to fluctuations in symptoms, it is difficult to adapt consistently to the care recipient's limitations and personality changes and to adjust to living together accordingly; for the caregiver, uncertainties and doubts arise again and again regarding their own behavior and attitudes toward the care recipient.
- The cognitive and personality changes associated with dementia are grieved in a way similar to grieving the loss of an ill partner or parent: The intensity and depth of this "anticipatory grief" is comparable to grieving the death of a loved one and represents considerable emotional burden.
- For caregiving within a marriage, the healthy spouse must take on new roles and functions, which can lead to persistent overload: Prospects for joint planning of life together in late adulthood must be abandoned or reconsidered.
- Adult children must make decisions for their now dependent parent with dementia: Role reversal and parentification of the children occur.
- Caring for a family member is not only based on emotional attachment and closeness, but can also be motivated by feelings of obligation or gratitude, moral or familial norms, (presumed) expectations of other family members, or the social environment. This can lead to the experience of burden if the caregivers do not perceive the expected gratitude from the family member with dementia or other family members and if conflicts arise in the caregiving situation.

- Fantasies of detachment from the partner or the parent who has now become a stranger, or the desire for their death as a liberation from the burdensome caregiving situation can elicit considerable feelings of guilt.

1.3 Models and Predictors for Burden and Coping With Caregiving

Pearlin's stress model (Pearlin et al., 1990) addresses and gives structure to some of these complex challenges that family caregivers face. On the one hand, this model describes primary stressors in caregiving, such as sociodemographic variables, type of care arrangement, and development of care. These are further categorized into objective (e.g., cognitive status, everyday-life skills, problem behaviors) and subjective (overburden, loss of relationship quality, appraisal of stress) stressors. On the other hand, *secondary stressors* are defined, which are subdivided into role stressors (familial tasks, occupation) and intra-psychological stressors (coping and self-esteem, loss of self). Additionally, the *consequences* (health, well-being, taking on a new role, use of healthcare services) stemming from those demands, as well as the caregivers' *resources* (coping with problems and emotions, finding meaning in caregiving, and social support), are taken into consideration. In section 1.3.1, the most important of the above-mentioned stress-related and influential factors are described in detail.

1.3.1 Problem Behavior as Well as Noncognitive Symptoms and Neuropsychiatric Disorders

A high level of stress can be observed in caregivers when there is an increase in problem behavior as well as in noncognitive neuropsychiatric disorders such as anxiety, lack of drive, apathy, or restlessness. Behavioral abnormalities play a crucial role in the caregiver's well-being and early nursing-home placement (Coen et al., 2002; Perren et al., 2006). They are of greater importance than the cognitive and functional impairments in the person with dementia (Perren et al., 2006), the number of caregiving tasks, as well as the duration of care (Fauth & Gibbons, 2014). The more frequently behavioral problems occur and the higher their severity is, the lower the well-being of the family caregiver (Perren et al., 2006). An increase in behavioral symptoms leads to increased stress experience and deterioration of the caregiver's health (Hooker et al., 2002). In addition, behavioral disorders also have a negative effect on the person with dementia's well-being (Haupt et al., 2000; Hurt et al., 2008). Furthermore, the challenging behavior also changes the quality of the relationship between caregivers and care recipients and can lead to depressive mood for caregivers (Schoenmakers et al., 2010).

1.3.2 Grief and Family Caregivers' Experience of Loss

The experience of grief in informal caregivers commences long before the actual death of the person with dementia (Cheung et al., 2018). This phenomenon is referred to as *anticipatory grief* (Lindemann, 1994) or *predeath grief* (Meuser & Marwit, 2001). The prevalence among family caregivers of people with dementia ranges from 47 % to 80 % (Dehpour & Koffman, 2023). The grief experienced is hardly different from grief after a close person's death (Meuser et al., 2004). Family members who stated that they did not grieve nevertheless expressed strong feelings of loss when they talked about the person with dementia, even though they did not classify their emotions as grief. Due to the specific dementia symptoms, family members often have difficulty naming the experience of loss, because the person with dementia still physically participates in life, while their personality increasingly changes. Thus, predeath grief in dementia is a distinctive type of grief characterized by compound serial losses, including the loss of intimacy and companionship, personal freedom, and social or occupational opportunities: Moreover, role identity separates and emotionally disconnects the caregiver from the still physically present person with dementia (Dehpour & Koffman, 2023). The cause of such a grief reaction can be understood in the context of attachment theory models (Bowlby, 1977). People form attachments based on their desire for protection and security. When such an attachment is threatened or broken by death, illness, or other critical life events, a grieving process occurs. Due to the progressive course of dementia, this adaptation process persists and represents an extreme emotional burden for the family member (Dempsey & Baago, 1998). Ambivalence with feelings of hope and resignation arises. This ambiguity regarding loss can also lead to family members not openly admitting their grief, making them less likely to want to make use of outside help and/or support (Dempsey & Baago, 1998; Sanders et al., 2007). Moreover, the necessary grieving process is complicated by the lack of recognition in the environment. The experienced feelings of shame, embarrassment, anger, and fury cannot be communicated. The lack of exchange in this respect can lead to social withdrawal (Frank, 2008) and avoidance of openly talking about grief (Walker et al., 1995).

Holley and Mast (2009) showed that the intensity of family caregivers' experienced grief can be considered as one of the most important and constant predictors of burden. Accordingly, caregivers experiencing a higher level of grief reported lower well-being and higher caregiver burden (Cheung et al., 2018) as well as higher perceived stress (Kobiske et al., 2019). Although predeath grief and caregiver burden share risk factors (later stage of dementia, behavioral problems of the person with dementia, and primary caregiving role), there are also risk factors unique to predeath grief, namely a younger age of the person with dementia, lower educational attainment of caregivers, and being a spousal caregiver (Liew et al., 2019).

The extent to which family caregivers are able to cope with and adapt to relationship and role changes and/or losses depends largely on how caregivers deal with their grief over the experienced losses (Kasl-Godley, 2003). Results of some studies suggest that adequately dealing with the experienced losses positively influences how dementia caregivers cope with both caregiving and grief after the person with dementia's death (Kasl-Godley, 2003). Those who do not deal with such losses prior to the death of their family member with dementia showed higher depression and anxiety scores as well as complicated grief symptoms after the death (Hebert et al., 2006). Research results from Boerner et al. (2004) and Hebert and Schulz (2006) showed that many family caregivers experience difficult and, to some extent, long-lasting grief. One year after the person with dementia's death, 30 % of family caregivers fulfilled the criteria for a depressive disorder, and 20 % fulfilled the criteria for complicated grief (Hebert & Schulz, 2006).

In this context, it should be noted that a strained relationship with the person with dementia before dementia onset has been identified as a fundamental predictor of psychological impairment in caregivers. Williamson and Shaffer (2000) showed that dementia family caregivers were less depressed and were less aggressive, impulsive, and impatient in caregiving situations if the relationship before taking on the caregiver role was characterized by mutual respect for each other's needs.

1.3.3 Experiencing and Witnessing Changes in the Care Recipient due to Dementia

The caregiver's perception of the care recipient's suffering substantially impacts the caregiver's experience of burden and depression (Huang, 2022; Schulz et al., 2017). Especially when the caregiver sees no possibility in positively influencing the relative with dementia's emotional state, sympathizing with and witnessing their family member suffering presents a heavy burden (Monin & Schulz, 2009).

1.3.4 Role Changes and Taking on New Roles

The loss of autonomy and the personality changes mostly associated with dementia are experienced by healthy spouses as a massive change in their relationship because usual behavior patterns in the relationship are no longer reacted to in a familiar way by the person with dementia (Clark et al., 2019). The partner's dementia thus disturbs the existing role allocation within a generally long-lasting marital relationship. The healthy partner's assumption of new roles often contributes to their overload (Välimäki et al., 2012). The redefinition of marital identity, in which both the ill and healthy partners take on new roles, can be complicated because dementia symptoms often fluctuate, thus making it more difficult to come to terms with the adapting process. Sometimes, dementia symptoms are denied, or their severity is misconceived in order to withstand the tension between strangeness and familiarity. These burdensome aspects of the relationship with the ill partner or parent can lead to denial about dementia (Clark et al., 2019). However, an adaptation of family life to the disease cannot be achieved in this case: Family caregivers react inadequately to the cognitive and behavioral impairments, and the person with dementia will be overtaxed with trying to behave like a healthy person. For adult children, role reversal and parentification occur, which can have considerable potential for conflict for both sides and require the caregiving children to adapt substantially (Välimäki et al., 2012).

Therefore, it is understandable that caregivers are extremely burdened by the changes in the relationship (Enright et al., 2020) and are more likely to give up home care and move their family member to a nursing home. For example, the increasing loss of knowledge of their own identity and the accumulation of situations when they no longer recognize their family members is particularly burdensome and thus often associated with the decision for nursing-home placement (Annerstedt et al., 2000).

1.3.5 Social Isolation and Insufficient Social Support

Another major burden is the social isolation many caregivers fall into while providing care. On the one hand, this occurs due to reduced time and organizational possibilities for socializing, and, on the other hand, because friends and close relatives often withdraw themselves (Liu et al., 2021; Wawrziczny et al., 2017). Although dementia has become increasingly less taboo in recent years, many caregivers still report social exclusion from preexisting networks. Lack of knowledge and uncertainty regarding how one should deal with the person with dementia are often responsible for this reaction from the social environment (Wawrziczny et al., 2017). The experience of burden is especially pronounced when caregivers receive unsatisfactory and insufficient professional support (Lee et al., 2022; Xu et al., 2021).

Furthermore, the COVID-19 pandemic increased social isolation and, therefore, the burden of caregivers of a person who is at high risk for severe COVID-19 disease and mortality. Thus, the importance of social support and access to social resources for the caregivers' well-being became even more evident (Cohen et al., 2020). Moreover, the COVID-19 pandemic further highlights the importance of access to *remote* forms of therapy, especially for family caregivers.

1.4 Family Caregivers' Coping Strategies

Family members of persons with dementia use various strategies to cope with the stressful care situation, and these strategies vary from individual to individual. Studies conclude that strategies such as active problem solving, searching for information, or positive reassessment and acceptance have a stress-reducing effect (Gilhooly et al., 2016). Due to the course of disease progression in dementia, many problems faced by caregivers cannot be changed, despite caregivers' greatest efforts. Therefore, successful coping includes the ability to recognize one's own limits and strengths, to ask for help, and to learn to accept the disease and its consequences (Kneebone & Martin, 2003). One's attitude toward the caregiver role also affects the level of experienced burden. Finding meaning or personal growth in caregiving eases coping (McLennon et al., 2011). Subjective appraisals also affect whether objective stress factors, especially disease-related behavioral changes, are experienced as strenuous and exhausting. Furthermore, given the same level of objective difficulties, the subjective burden experience depends on the caregiver's conviction on whether they have the situation under control and are able to cope with the situation by their own efforts. Various studies point to the importance of self-efficacy beliefs for caregiver burden. Belief in one's own self-efficacy with respect to dealing with behavioral problems and the ability to control anger-generating thoughts reduces stress and especially anxiety and depressive symptoms (Lopez et al., 2012; Nogáles-González et al., 2015). In contrast, avoidance strategies such as wishful thinking, resignation, or passive complaining can lead to depressive symptoms (Gilhooly et al., 2016). Moreover, the availability of social support and positively rated social contacts can provide relief (Atienza et al., 2001).

1.5 Positive Aspects of Caregiving

Besides the burden of caregiving, a substantial proportion of family caregivers report positive experiences through providing care, such as increased intimacy with the care recipient, strengthening of self-esteem, personal growth, a sense of purpose, and the feeling that providing care is worthwhile (Cabote et al., 2015). Family caregivers who could find important meaning or personal purpose in providing care showed fewer depressive symptoms and had higher self-esteem, and this positive appraisal was not related to objective stressors of providing care (Noonan & Tennstedt, 1997). These positive aspects of caregiving can thus compensate for burden, reduce depression, and increase the caregiver's well-being (Pinquart & Sörensen, 2004; Wu et al., 2022). In addition, despite changes and burden, closeness and intimacy to the care recipient is usually preserved and enables continuous, valuable shared experiences (Bjørge et al., 2019).

2
Need for and Effectiveness of Psychosocial Interventions

This chapter presents the need and requirements for helpful family caregiver interventions, the current state of research regarding specific intervention studies, as well as recommendations for family dementia caregiver interventions that are based on these research findings.

2.1 Need for Helpful Family Caregiver Interventions

The results of numerous studies indicate that the utilization of professional support (such as day care, outpatient home care) reduces caregiver burden and contributes to a longer stay at home for the person with dementia (Eska et al., 2013; Vandepitte et al., 2016). Paradoxically, however, despite the high need for professional assistance, there is relatively low usage of the available support (Brodaty et al., 2005; Lamura et al., 2006; Røsvik et al., 2020). In a cross-sectional study with 170 family caregivers, less than half of the family caregivers (42 %) used professional help (Rother & Wilz, 2010). Family members of people with dementia usually hesitate for a long time until they seek outside assistance (Neville et al., 2015) and many caregivers feel ashamed to ask for or accept help (Winslow, 2003).

Acquiring information on available support may be difficult for family caregivers due to their social isolation. Many family caregivers do not have adequate information about dementia, treatment options, and available support services. Generally, family members are often too stressed to seek help and report that they do not have the time to gather information. Some also criticize that the information for the service providers is too extensive, making it difficult to have an overview and compare them (Bieber et al., 2019; Stephan et al., 2018). In a review

Bieber et al. (2019) showed the following main concerns of caregivers: attitudes toward services, financial aspects, burden and stress, behavioral problems of the person with dementia, and worries about restriction of one's own independence.

In the case of out-of-home services, especially in rural areas, there may also be concerns regarding others' reactions. Moreover family caregivers could be afraid that information shared in caregiver groups will not be treated confidentially (Morgan et al., 2002). Additional important psychological barriers are family caregivers' worries about alienation or distancing themselves from the person with dementia, or fear that, for example, a day-care center visit could increase concern for the well-being of the person with dementia or cause severe unrest (Schacke & Zank, 1998).

For home services, caregivers complain about intrusion of privacy. They do not want to have a stranger in their household, under whose observation they might feel controlled (Roelands et al., 2008). The rejection of help by the person with dementia, the lack of the caregivers' acceptance of professional assistance, as well as feelings of guilt and obligation are also discussed as important barriers (Grässel et al., 2010).

The selected findings show that the decision-making process regarding whether and which type of professional assistance is utilized is complex and particularly dependent on individual appraisals of the situation. Psychological interventions for prevention and reduction of burden-related secondary diseases for dementia caregivers should thus specifically take these mental barriers into account. The modification of obstructive attitudes toward utilization of support (changing dysfunctional thoughts) and the encouragement of acceptance and utilization of relieving assistance offers are therefore considered essential objectives of professional family caregiver interventions.

2.2 Demands for Helpful Family Caregiver Interventions

In a review of 34 studies Bressan et al. (2020) classified the needs of family caregivers into four themes: being supported by formal services and emotionally, receiving accessible and personalized information, being trained and educated to manage changes, and finding a balance to deal with changes in their lives and time for themselves. Taking these topics into account, as well as the challenges of dementia caregiving presented in Chapter 1, interventions should include the following aspects:

- imparting knowledge on dementia, financial and legal issues, and support services;
- modifying the appraisal of symptoms to promote understanding and acceptance of the disease;
- developing strategies for dealing with behavioral problems and promoting problem-solving skills;
- coping with and accepting the new role;
- supporting the caregiver in processing the change of the relationship and disease-related losses, and developing strategies for dealing with stressful emotions such as grief, anger, fury, guilt, shame, anxiety, and depression;
- improving the perception of stress limits and encouraging self-care and consideration of one's own needs;
- identifying dysfunctional thoughts and schemes regarding one's own caregiving abilities, perfectionism in caregiving, and assumption of responsibility;
- removing barriers to and promoting utilization of professional and informal support;
- encouraging helpful, positive family relationships as well as shared positive activities with the person with dementia.

Thus, a wide range of intervention strategies is required in order to provide adequate support for the above-mentioned problem areas. A sole focus on managing objective stressors is overly simplistic as it ignores the psychopathological (e.g., dysfunctional thoughts, activity restriction, and experiential avoidance) as well as salutogenetic factors (e.g., utilizing the available psychosocial resources) that lead to caregivers' subjective appraisal of caregiving as either burdensome or manageable (see Chapter 1).

2.3 CBT-Based Caregiver Interventions: Content, Evaluation, and Recommendations

Among the numerous interventions for family caregivers of people with dementia, cognitive behavioral therapy (CBT) has been found to be particularly effective on depression, anxiety, and burden. However, on other outcomes such as physical health, quality of life, or stress, effects of CBT were not consistent (Cheng et al., 2019; Gallagher-Thompson & Coon, 2007; Hopkinson et al., 2019; Verreault et al., 2021). Following a detailed description and analyses of these single studies, the meta-analysis by Cheng et al. (2019) presented a differentiated overview.

An explanation of the inconsistency of CBT yielding effects on a wider range of outcomes could be that only a few caregiver intervention studies implemented a comprehensive CBT approach and used sound evaluation methods. The analysis of the type and frequency of intervention methods used in previous studies shows that, to date, the majority of studies focused solely on only a part of the burden and problem areas, using a limited repertoire of intervention strategies (Kurz & Wilz, 2011). The most frequently used strategies were ones to improve problem-solving skills, followed by imparting knowledge, and, third, guidance for self-care. Interventions focused much less often on expanding the support network, modification of dysfunctional thoughts, emotion regulation, or coping with loss and grief (Kurz & Wilz, 2011).

Few caregiver intervention studies have focused on changing dysfunctional cognitions, although this focus represents one of the most efficient cognitive-behavioral strategies, particularly for treating depressive symptoms. Such cognitions can include, for example, thoughts reflecting over-protectiveness (e.g., not letting the care recipient do things of which they are capable out of a fear that they will fail) or dysfunctional thoughts, which prohibit receipt of professional or informal support. One important objective of these effective interventions is to encourage caregivers to think more adaptively and to develop more realistic beliefs and goals that facilitate their everyday coping with caregiving demands and their own self-care. The benefits of changing dysfunctional thoughts have been demonstrated with respect to caregivers' depressive symptoms (Losada et al., 2011) and anxiety (Vernooij-Dassen et al., 2011).

In the following paragraphs a selection of studies with a comprehensive cognitive-behavioral intervention approach will be described in more detail.

Losada et al. (2011) conceptualized a 12-hour group program, in which primarily cognitive restructuring and pleasant activity scheduling were used as intervention methods. The family caregivers in the intervention group benefited in terms of reduced depressive symptoms, increased pleasant activities, and a decline in dysfunctional thoughts, compared to the untreated control group.

In the study by (Coon et al., 2003), two different treatment concepts were compared. In the anger management group, the intervention methods were frustration management, relaxation skills, positive self-instruction, self-observation of dysfunctional thoughts, as well as social competence training and role-playing within the framework of 10 group sessions. In the depression management group, the relationship between mood and positive activities was explained, a self-change plan was developed, and individual goals were defined. Moreover, the therapeutic work involved encouraging positive activities and problem-solving skills with a focus on cognitive interventions (10 group sessions). Both intervention concepts showed positive effects in terms of reductions in depressive symptoms, hostility, and anger, compared to the waiting-list control group.

Gallagher-Thompson et al.'s (2000) study also compared two intervention groups with 10 group sessions each. In the group, increasing life satisfaction, the intervention focused on observing the relationship between positive activities and mood, promoting positive activities, developing a self-change plan, and on individual goals. In the increasing problem-solving group, the intervention comprised strategies for improving problem-solving skills, stress management, emotion regulation, and differentiation between changeable and unchangeable situations. The comparison with the waiting-list condition showed an improvement in depressive symptoms only for the increasing life satisfaction group. However, an increase in action-related coping strategies was found for both intervention groups.

In a follow-up study, the Gallagher-Thompson et al. (2003) research group compared a CBT-based group therapy with traditional supportive family caregiver groups. Several CBT techniques were implemented: stress management, relaxation techniques, realistic evaluations of the person with dementia's behavior, social competence training, promotion of positive activities, and creation of a self-change plan. The CBT group showed a decrease in depressive symptoms and an increase in positive coping strategies in comparison to the support group.

An extension of this approach was investigated in a follow-up study (Gallagher-Thompson et al., 2008). Within 13 to 16 weekly group sessions, a wide range of CBT strategies were used: psychoeducation, dealing with behavioral abnormalities, problem solving, role-play, homework, changing dysfunctional thoughts, promoting social competence, positive activities and shared activities with the person with dementia, promoting self-care, relaxation training, imparting professional support services, as well as planning for the future regarding the person with dementia's needs. The results showed reductions in depressive symptoms and in general caregiving-related experienced stress. Moreover, more caregiving-related skills were reported, and the caregivers rated the CBT group as more helpful than the minimal telephone-based support that the control group received.

In the REACH II study Belle et al. (2006) evaluated a multicomponent intervention including education, skills to manage problem behaviors, social support, cognitive strategies, and strategies for enhancing healthy behaviors and managing stress. The intervention consisted of 12 in-home and telephone sessions over a period of 6 months. The results showed greater improvement in quality of life (using a composite score including the outcomes depression, burden, self-care, social support, and care recipient problem behaviors) for Hispanic, Latino, and Caucasian caregivers of the intervention group compared to a control group with minimal support.

In the study of Losada et al. (2015) CBT and ACT (acceptance and commitment therapy) and a control group were compared. In the CBT group the intervention concept included cognitive restructuring, promoting social support, relaxation, and increasing pleasant activities. In the ACT group participants were encouraged to accept that aspects of the disease and the care situation cannot be changed. Participants learned how to manage negative emotions and cognitions in a more helpful way. Both intervention groups successfully reduced dementia caregivers' depressive symptomatology, anxiety, dysfunctional thoughts, and increased their leisure activities at postintervention. Experiential avoidance was only reduced in the ACT group and follow-up effects were only found for depression in the CBT group.

Regarding the findings of the described meta-analyses and intervention studies, the following recommendations should be considered: Effective interventions actively include family members by using behavioral exercises, role-play, and exercises for dealing with the person with dementia. Accordingly, family-related interventions that included additional family members and encouraged empathic communication showed positive effects. Further specific cognitive-behavioral interventions such as stress management, emotion regulation, and cognitive interventions were able to yield positive results. It is important to enable caregivers of people with dementia to develop more adaptive and realistic beliefs and goals that facilitate their coping with caregiving demands and encourage self-care. Moreover, because many aspects of the disease and the care situation cannot be changed, helping caregivers in managing and accepting the negative emotions and cognitions accompanying such burdensome experiences is another central objective of interventions (Wilz et al., 2018a).

2.3.1 Recommendations for the Timing and Duration of the Intervention

Although the meta-analyses of Hopkinson et al. (2019) could not find differences between lower numbers (less than eight) and higher numbers (greater than eight) of sessions, there could be stated some evidence that intensive and long-term interventions led to more sustainable effects (Cheng et al., 2019). For example, Mittelman et al.'s (2004) effective intervention concept consisted of an intensive support phase lasting 4 months with subsequent unlimited offers such as telephone counseling and family groups. Also, the only effective intervention of the REACH I study was characterized by a high number of sessions (52) and a long intervention period of 12 months (Eisdorfer et al., 2003). Accordingly, the positively evaluated REACH II intervention comprises a total of 12 sessions over a period of 6 months (Belle et al., 2006). In conclusion, family caregiver interventions should comprise not less than 10 sessions over a period of at least 3 months. Intervention periods lasting half a year or longer could be assessed as particularly effective (Töpfer et al., 2021).

2.3.2 Recommendations for Setting Conditions

Individual single-person interventions that were tailored to the caregivers' risk profiles using a case-formulation approach were able to achieve a high level of acceptance and good effectiveness (Márquez-González et al., 2020; Wilz et al., 2018b). Such individualized approaches are also of great importance because the personally specific problem situations and associated consequences for experience of burden can be taken into account (Cheng et al., 2019; Zarit et al., 2010).

Although several group concepts were proven to be effective, they pose a barrier to participation for a large proportion of family caregivers. In many cases, family caregivers are not mobile due to their own illnesses, cannot leave the person with dementia at home alone, or cannot take them to a group session due to their impairments. In addition, heavily burdened family caregivers with increased levels of depression and anxiety rarely participate in group interventions. Moreover, psychological barriers such as anxiety, inhibitions, or disappointing experiences are often the cause for nonparticipation in groups.

Therefore, in-home or remote interventions offer a large advantage (Wasilewski et al., 2017). Both settings are easier for family caregivers to integrate into their daily care routine, and these interventions guarantee better accessibility to the caregivers (Mohr et al., 2012). The advantage of home interventions is that they provide an insight into the daily care routines and the family life environment, thus allowing for individually suitable interventions to be selected.

Alternatively, video- or telephone-based intervention reaches a larger group of caregivers and represents an intervention procedure that can be implemented well in everyday practice. This form of support is particularly helpful for caregivers who are themselves ill, are not mobile, or do not have additional care support for the person with dementia. Furthermore, video or telephone support can better integrated into daily care routines, as no time is added for driving (Meichsner et al., 2019a).

Despite evidence suggesting that CBT via video or telephone (TEL-CBT) constitutes a promising alternative to face-to-face CBT (Jackson et al., 2016; Waller et al., 2017), only two studies have so far directly compared TEL-CBT and F2F-CBT (face-to-face CBT) for family caregivers of people with dementia. Glueckauf et al. (2012) found in a pilot study with 11 caregivers, that TEL-CBT ($n=6$) and F2F-CBT ($n=5$) did not significantly differ on subjective burden, assistance support, physical symptoms, and depression. Both modes of delivery yielded comparable effect sizes in the low to moderate range. Töpfer et al. (2023) showed, that TEL-CBT yielded significantly better physical health ($d=0.27$) and coping with daily hassles (*d* = 0.38) at posttest compared to F2F-CBT. Therapist competence, acceptability, and outcomes at follow-up did not differ between TEL-CBT and F2F-CBT.

2.4 Concept and Evaluation of the Tele.TAnDem Intervention

The Tele.TAnDem manual (teletherapy for family caregivers of people with dementia [Therapeutische Unterstützung für pflegende Angehörige von Menschen mit Demenz. Das Tele.TAnDem-Behandlungsprogramm], Wilz et al., 2015) was developed to address the extremely challenging situation of family caregivers of people with dementia. It is predicated on the idea of using evidence-based psychotherapeutic strategies to support family caregivers. The theoretical approach is CBT and further incorporates principles of ACT and includes therefore cognitive, behavioral, problem-solving, emotion-regulation, acceptance, and resource-activation interventions. As CBT aims to guide individuals to develop both cognitive and behavioral skills for coping with stressful and difficult situations, these features make CBT particularly appropriate for application in the complex and demanding context of family caregiving.

Accordingly, it is an important objective of interventions to enable caregivers to develop more adaptive and realistic beliefs and goals that facilitate their coping with caregiving demands and to encourage self-care. The additional use of ACT-based elements can support family caregivers in a much stronger way than traditional CBT alone, especially with respect to adopting a nonjudgmental and more accepting approach and mindset. Since many aspects of the disease and the caregiving situation cannot be changed, helping caregivers in managing and accepting the negative emotions and cognitions accompanying such a difficult experience (e.g., anger, grief, shame, guilt, anxiety, and depression) is a central objective of the interventions.

2.4.1 Overview of the Content of the Intervention Concept

While the therapy concept is manualized on the one hand, providing therapists with detailed information and material on different modules, it also accounts for the importance of individually tailored treatment by guiding therapists to use and combine the modules according to the individual needs and therapy goals of the respective caregiver.

These modules will comprise the following:
1. Content, setting, procedure, and overview of intervention strategies: Specific aspects of various setting conditions, the structure of the therapy process, and an overview of the therapeutic strategies are presented.
2. First session and building a therapeutical relationship: Contents are how to structure the first session and creating the therapeutic alliance over the whole therapy process.
3. Changing dysfunctional cognitions: Through Socratic dialogue, guided discovery, and the ABC model (adverse event, beliefs, consequences) (Ellis, 1977), the therapist and caregiver work out alternative and more helpful thoughts and appraisals as well as possibilities to test and transfer these alternative thoughts in real life.
4. Coping with challenging behavior of the care recipient, strengthening problem-solving abilities: Through behavior analyses and problem-solving training, clients are instructed and supported in their individual problem-solving process.
5. Stress management and emotion-regulation strategies: Accepting emotions such as anger as a normal emotion, finding distance to stressful emotions in order to analyze situations, developing emotion-regulation strategies, working on acceptance and the general tension level.
6. Self-care, creating value-based activities: Potential incentives are to be increased through the following mechanism – description of the link between positive activities and mood by means of a weekly diary, lists of health-promoting activities, planning of activities, and promoting their implementation. Furthermore, accepting negative feelings such as guilty conscience toward the care recipient while moving toward undertaking value-based activities.
7. Coping with change, grief, and loss: Central topics are coping with changes caused by the disease, the loss of the personal relationship, and resulting feelings of grief. Emotion-based coping strategies, acceptance of the illness and its resulting changes, as well as experiences of loss are discussed.
8. Increasing the use of informal and professional support in caregiving: Possibilities of professional and informal help are addressed. The process of allow-

ing and accepting help is discussed, using cognitive restructuring and behavior experiments.
9. Limits of caregiving: Identification and consequences for when caregivers reach their breaking point or maximum stress load in caregiving. Support during nursing-home placement: decision for/against, preparations, and transition phase.
10. Evaluation: Achieved changes and goals are summarized, stimulating long-term transfer and plans for the future are discussed.

2.4.2 Number of Sessions, Duration, and Setting Conditions of the Intervention Concept

The intervention consists of 12 (50-minute) therapeutic sessions of individual CBT provided by trained psychotherapists, counselors, or social workers within 6 months. The first four sessions take place at weekly intervals, six further sessions follow at biweekly intervals, and the two last sessions at monthly intervals. However, the concept can also be implemented more flexibly and shortened to fewer sessions, supplemented with booster sessions, or even extended over more sessions continuously over a longer time.

It is a special feature of the therapy manual that it can be (besides individual face-to-face or video sessions) delivered successfully via telephone or online. Since many family caregivers of people with dementia are often unable to attend face-to-face sessions because they cannot leave the care recipient alone, have physical constraints, or reside in rural areas with poor infrastructure, delivering the intervention remotely increases accessibility.

The remote verbal contact and the support of the therapist were rated as very positive by the majority of the caregivers, with an emphasis on the therapists' high levels of empathy, respectful attitudes, preparation for the sessions, and high levels of expertise. Eighty-one percent of the caregivers stated that their expectations of the intervention were "fully" or "predominantly" fulfilled, and 91% would recommend the intervention to other people. The telephone setting was rated by 72% of participants as very good, and by 27% as good (Wilz et al., 2011; Wilz et al., 2018b).

2.4.3 Tele.TAnDem Evaluation Results

The therapy manual is an evidence-based intervention, evaluated in four separate randomized-controlled trials supporting its short-term and long-term benefits. In all trials the psychotherapeutic intervention was administrated by clinically experienced psychologists who were trained in CBT (either board-certified or in advanced stages of training). The therapists had extensive knowledge on dementia, on dealing with behavioral problems, and in terms of the specific caregiving situation. The therapy sessions were supervised by the project director and external supervisors. To ensure and evaluate treatment integrity, all therapy sessions were recorded, and their therapeutic quality was reviewed using a rating system by external, trained raters (Schinköthe & Wilz, 2014).

The therapy manual has been evaluated, applied, and compared in different settings such as individual face-to-face sessions, via telephone, and online (Meichsner et al., 2019a; Töpfer et al., 2022, 2023; Wilz et al., 2018a).

The short-term Tele.TAnDem intervention with seven sessions has been compared to a control group receiving progressive muscle relaxation (PMR) and an untreated control group receiving usual care (Wilz & Soellner, 2016). Tele.TAnDem significantly improved emotional well-being (compared to the PMR and control group) and decreased body complaints (compared to the control group) posttreatment.

The evaluation of goal attainment yielded that more than two thirds of the intervention group participants achieved complete or partial goal attainment (Wilz et al., 2011). At 6-month follow-up, participants who had received Tele.TAnDem reported significantly fewer depressive symptoms (compared to the PMR group) and improved perceived health (compared to the control group). Long-term effects 2 years after treatment were found for emotional well-being, health status, bodily complaints, and quality of life (Wilz et al., 2017).

The Tele.TAnDem intervention was subsequently extended as participants evaluated the short-term intervention as helpful but the number of sessions as too few and the duration of the intervention as too short (Wilz & Soellner, 2016). The extended intervention, consisting of twelve 50-minute sessions over the course of 6 months, showed treatment effects on well-being, depression, body complaints, coping with the care situation, and coping with the behavior of the care recipient at posttest compared to usual care. The effects on well-being and coping maintained at 6-month follow-up (Wilz et al., 2018a).

Furthermore, quality of life was significantly improved in the domains of psychological health, physical health, and overall quality of life at posttest (Meichsner et al., 2019b). Tele.TAnDem also significantly increased dementia caregivers' utilization of psychosocial resources related to well-being and coping with daily hassles following the intervention (Töpfer & Wilz, 2018) and reduced the burden due to predeath grief until 6 months after treatment (Meichsner & Wilz, 2018).

Nearly all participants reported meaningful improvements regarding their personal goals (Wilz et al., 2018b). The majority of caregivers (69.9 %) stated full or partial goal attainment, 24.1 % could achieve stabilization, only 3.6 % reported a worsening of their problem situation, and 2.4 % reported overachievement of their goals (Wilz et al., 2018b).

In one of the few studies investigating mediating mechanisms of dementia caregiver interventions, Töpfer and Wilz (2021) provided evidence that utilization of resources related to well-being and coping mediated the effects of the extended Tele.TAnDem intervention on caregivers' quality of life at posttest and 6-month follow-up.

In the Tele.TAnDem online study the intervention was delivered via individualized written email contact (eight sessions). The results showed enhanced resource realization for well-being, reduced care-related grief, and improved well-being for the intervention group (Meichsner et al., 2019a).

Finally, and importantly, the therapy manual is also successful in buffering detrimental effects of caregiving even in the long term. Caregivers in the Tele.TAnDem intervention group reported significantly lower caregiver burden, higher quality of life regarding social relationships, and improved coping with behavior problems of the person with dementia 2.5 years postintervention (Töpfer et al., 2021).

In sum, in order to therapeutically fulfill the complex, and especially emotional burden that family caregivers report, interventions based on cognitive-behavioral psychotherapy approaches should therefore be considered as suitable due to their proven effectiveness and their variety of methods (Cheng et al., 2019).

Furthermore, besides all these useful intervention strategies, the concepts should be overall based on resource orientation, strengthening competence, and confidence and self-esteem of the caregivers through on the one hand specific intervention strategies and on the other hand through a respectful and empathic therapeutic relationship (Theurer & Wilz, 2022; Wrede et al., 2023).

3 Helpful Information on Dementia and Caregiving-Specific Issues for Family Caregivers

Family caregivers often have special dementia-specific, caregiving-specific, and legal questions, e.g., regarding symptoms, course of the illness, medication, and financing of care services or support. Therefore, the therapist should have knowledge about the disease and the organization of care. However, the therapy sessions do not cover any medical, care-related, or financial or legal advice in the narrower sense. The therapist is usually not specifically trained for this task and the limited duration of the therapy sessions is necessary for the application of the therapeutic interventions. However, the therapist should show the family caregivers how they can obtain further information. The International Alzheimer's Society (Alzheimer's Association, 2022), the respective national and regional Alzheimer's societies, and special information or counselling centers can provide such information and advice. The therapy thus considers itself as a door opener and mediator to other competent centers with respect to dementia and care-specific questions. This chapter provides an overview of issues commonly raised by family caregivers.

3.1 Illness-Specific Topics

3.1.1 Dementia Diagnosis

At the beginning and sometimes during the later course of therapy, it is important to provide the family caregivers with an understandable picture of the symptoms of dementia. Family caregivers often do not know the exact diagnosis or know little about the course of the symptoms, so acquiring relevant knowledge can lead to more understanding and acceptance of the illness. The use of technical terms should be avoided, and the impartment of specialist knowledge should be adapted to the family caregiver's individual comprehension level.

Alzheimer's disease is the most common form of dementia (approx. 60–90 %). In contrast, vascular dementia (approx. 20 %) and dementia associated with other diseases (less than 10 %) are less common (American Psychiatric Association, 2013). However, it is often not possible to clearly distinguish between the forms of dementia in psychotherapeutic sessions with the family caregivers. If the diagnosis is unclear for the family caregivers, it can be helpful to be informed about the diagnosis and the symptoms during a consultation with the physician treating their family member with dementia. Concerning the possible causes of the dementia syndrome, which can be very diverse and are relevant for the treatment of the person with dementia, the family caregivers should also seek a consultation with the physician.

If there is only a suspicion of dementia, a careful diagnosis should be carried out in an appropriate clinic or by a specialist.

First, the therapist can ask the family caregivers to describe the changes, problems, and abnormalities in their family member with dementia. Based on these descriptions, the symptoms of dementia can be individually identified, named, and classified so that the family caregiver can understand the dementia syndrome and classify daily symptoms.

In this context, a short definition of dementia can be given: According to the *Diagnostic and Statistical Manual of Mental Disorders* (5th ed.: *DSM-5*; American Psychiatric Association, 2013), dementia belongs to the category of neurocognitive disorders (NCD). The term NCD includes disorders that are mainly characterized by acquired deficits in cognitive function, for example: impairments in memory, thinking, orientation, perception, arithmetic, learning, language, judgment, and decision-making ability. In addition to cognitive impairments, there are changes in emotion regulation (e.g., anxiety, impulsiveness, aggressive behavior), social behavior (e.g., changes in manners), or motivation (e.g., lack of drive, lack of interest).

The classification of dementia according to *DSM-5* (American Psychiatric Association, 2013) is summarized in Box 1.

Box 1. Summary of the classification according to *DSM-5*

- Delirium
- Mild neurocognitive disorder
- Major neurocognitive disorder

"Mild neurocognitive disorder" is characterized by moderate cognitive decline, no impairment of independence, and is not due to delirium or other mental disorders. "Major neurocognitive disorder" is characterized by significant cognitive decline, impairment of independence, and is not due to delirium or other mental disorders.

Psychoeducation 1 illustrates how the therapist can explain these essential aspects of dementia in simple language.

Psychoeducation 1. Symptom presentation

> Dementia is a disease in which fewer and fewer brain cells function properly. It usually occurs only in old age. Not only is the ability to remember lost, but over time everyday activities can no longer be carried out. Other symptoms of dementia include repeating questions and behaviors, disorientation (e.g., a person with dementia gets lost in familiar places, is not sure of the time, date, and time of year, does not know where they are), loss of ability to follow cues, to make reasonable judgments and decisions, and to pay attention to personal safety, hygiene, and nutrition. Changes in personality and behavior also happen regularly (e.g., restlessness, anxiety, aggressive behavior).

3.1.2 Course of the Illness

It is important for the therapist to be sensitive and empathetic while talking about the progressive course of the illness with the family caregivers since this information is often associated with great fears and worries about the future. It is very important to inform the family caregivers that the symptoms can vary greatly from person to person. This depends on the respective form of dementia and the causes, but also on the person with dementia's individual resources. Therefore, the duration of caregiving can vary greatly and cover a long period of time (life expectancy 5–10 years following diagnosis).

How the course of the illness can be conveyed to the family caregivers is summarized in Psychoeducation 2. The example of Alzheimer's dementia is used since it occurs most frequently.

Psychoeducation 2. The course of Alzheimer's dementia

> Mild stage of dementia (2–4 years):
>
> At this stage, persons affected can usually still carry out their everyday tasks without extensive support from their family caregivers. However, the family caregivers notice changes and symptoms, possibly without being able to clearly classify them. After the diagnosis, family caregivers often say: "He changed 2 to 3 years ago, but I would never have thought of dementia, he simply withdrew a bit and sometimes behaved differently – but dementia?" Family caregivers often suspect depression, since persons affected with depression often show a loss of drive and low spirits, which can be related to experiencing an increasing loss of abilities.
>
> For the somewhat distant social environment, i.e., neighbors or family members who reside far away, the person with dementia usually still appears "normal" and "inconspicuous." This can give the impression that there are either no or hardly any impairments. Moreover, many people with dementia often do not talk about their problems (e.g., forgetfulness) and want to obscure their loss of abilities. However, by asking questions and careful observation, difficulties in finding words, and deficits in organizing or planning actions or other everyday tasks often become clear. At this stage, there are often fears, insecurities, and depressive symptoms. Another problem is that many of those affected do not want to go to the doctor on their own accord and avoid dealing with the disease.
>
> Moderate stage of dementia (2–10 years):
>
> Statistically, a moderate stage of dementia in Alzheimer's disease appears on average 3 years after the diagnosis. In this stage, those affected find it very difficult to retain new information and remember facts. Deficits in logical thinking, planning, and action, as well as in finding words and communication become evident for the environment. Many people suffering from dementia have difficulty orienting themselves spatially, especially in unfamiliar surroundings. In addition to the increasing cognitive deficits, behavioral changes and sometimes inappropri-

ate behavior become more apparent, which can cause more problems in public. For the family caregivers, these situations are usually experienced as unpleasant and are associated with feelings of shame, which is why certain situations are avoided. Particularly challenging, difficult behaviors are experienced by family caregivers as very burdensome. These behaviors include aggressive impulses, collecting and hoarding objects, wandering around, restlessness, as well as perpetually asking questions and following people around. Furthermore, nursing tasks increase, e.g., due to urinary incontinence. Those affected find it much more difficult to dress and to groom themselves. It is in this stage that people with dementia start to need extensive support from their family members and from professional services.

Severe stage of dementia (1–3 years):

People with Alzheimer's dementia reach the severe stage of dementia after an average of 6 years. It is important to note that this is a statistical measure; the course of the disease can vary greatly from person to person. At this stage, those affected are severely impaired in terms of their memory functions and everyday skills. Verbal communication with family members is possible only to a very limited extent or not at all. The inability to recognize the family caregiver and/or other family members is usually the most burdensome experience at this stage. However, people with dementia react to the emotional reactions of their counterparts. Since independent living is no longer possible, nursing and support tasks are prioritized. Round-the-clock support must often be ensured. This creates a high level of physical stress for the family caregivers, in addition to psychological stress. The day–night rhythm is disturbed in many of those affected, such that family caregivers are then usually severely impaired in their night's sleep. Eating becomes increasingly difficult. In addition to urinary incontinence, there can also be rectal incontinence, which is considerably burdensome for the family caregivers. The mobility of those affected (e.g., getting out of bed) is increasingly restricted, resulting in being bedridden. Care and nursing can no longer be provided by one family member alone. At this stage, at the latest, many family caregivers feel their limits in resilience.

Alzheimer's dementia usually progresses slowly, whereas vascular dementia often progresses incrementally or stepwise and can be accompanied by a temporary standstill or even slight improvements. Fluctuations in the symptoms and the abilities of everyday life can occur, are often difficult for the family caregivers to classify, and can lead to misjudgments regarding the disease. Therefore, the family caregivers should be informed that in the various stages there may be a temporary standstill or isolated short-term, nonlasting improvements in symptoms. Occasional confusion or doubts regarding the diagnosis can be counteracted in this way so that no irrational hope for improvement arises.

3.1.3 Problem Behaviors in Dementia

Problem behaviors occur in most people with dementia. These problematic behaviors are usually classified into the following symptom groups: affective symptoms, psychosis, hyperactivity (sometimes named agitation or psychomotor symptoms), and euphoria (van der Linde et al., 2014).

Family caregivers typically experience the following behaviors as very burdensome: aggressive behavior, screaming, restlessness, wandering around, constant following, socially inappropriate behavior, sexual disinhibition, hoarding, anxiety, depressive moods, apathy, hallucinations, and delusions. It is very relieving for family caregivers when they learn that these symptoms and behaviors are related to dementia and also occur in others living with dementia.

3.1.4 Causes of Problem Behaviors

Regardless of the form of dementia, those affected often feel overwhelmed due to the loss of cognitive functions and can no longer cope with everyday situations. Due to this stressful experience, they could react with irritation, fear, confusion, restlessness, and problem behaviors. Therefore, these behaviors should be primarily understood as a reaction to being overwhelmed and are functional for the persons with dementia in terms of emotion regulation, self-esteem stabilization, or securing autonomy (e.g., by obscuring deficits). However, these behaviors are usually perceived by family caregivers as inappropriate problem behaviors. It is, therefore, very important for family caregivers to develop an understanding of these reactions in therapy (see Chapter 9).

3.2 Medical Questions

Questions about medication, effects, and side effects should be referred to the treating physician since an assessment of these aspects from the therapist's point of view is not possible without specific medical qualifications and personal contact with the patient.

In addition to specific medical questions, family caregivers frequently address aspects of medical treatment. In this case, an appointment with the treating physician should also be recommended to clarify their concerns. The following aspects are frequently addressed by family caregivers:

- refusal by the person with dementia to visit a doctor;
- the person with dementia trivializing or denying their problems in front of the doctor;
- the unpleasant feeling of "showing" the person with dementia to the doctor;
- difficulty taking medication, e.g., due to problems swallowing or unreasonable fears;
- dissatisfaction with the medication;
- uncertainty when assessing the effects and side effects of the medication due to a lack of ability of the person with dementia to express themselves;
- problems with long waiting times or difficulties with finding appointments, especially in the case of working family caregivers;
- difficulty visiting specialists, e.g., dentist or gynecologist; and
- desire for more home visits.

For some of these problems, individual solutions can be developed using cognitive and emotion-related interventions as well as problem-solving strategies (e.g., relief when administering pills by using appropriate, supportive behavior, see Chapters 8–11).

3.3 Care-Related Questions

As the disease progresses, care and support issues become more and more important. Common care-related issues are summarized in Table 1.

Family caregivers often experience incontinence as particularly burdensome. Urinary incontinence, nocturnal urination, and – in advanced stages – rectal incontinence occur in many people with advanced dementia. In addition to financial and household problems, this also entails strong emotional stress for the family caregivers. On the subject of incontinence, reference should be made to good, easy-to-understand brochures, for example, from the Alzheimer's Association.

Questions often arise regarding the use of home care by licensed, skilled healthcare professionals, vacation care/respite care programs, or temporary care outpatient care services.

The greater the need for care is, the greater the need for practical and technical support. There are also other nursing aids that specified information or counselling centers can provide information about. Difficult ethical issues may arise with respect to hospice care, such as considering artificial feeding (e.g., through a nasogastric tube). The family caregivers should be offered the op-

Table 1. Caregiving-related issues

Area	Selected issues	Example
Nursing, caregiving, and housekeeping	Incontinence	Changing clothes and bedding nightly
	Nutrition	Eating/drinking too little or too much, difficulty ingesting
	Occupation	Finding no adequate activity for the person with dementia
Mobility	Getting up, walking, standing	Problems in lifting the person out of bed, fear of falling
	Leaving home	Refusal to go to day care, problems with public transport
Support	Coordination and organization	Problems with timing with outpatient services
	Environmental conditions	No shower in the bathroom, the bathtub can no longer be used, no adequate fixtures and fittings
	Aids	Improper incontinence products

portunity to discuss these topics in the therapy sessions and possibly go to counseling centers that are specialized in this.

3.4 Legal Questions

The symptoms of dementia lead to a changed perception of situations, limitations in the ability to make judgments, and deficits in assessing the consequences of one's actions. This can result in legal consequences for those affected and their families. In principle, family caregivers and persons with dementia should deal with these questions as early as possible. For many questions, such as power of attorney or living will, it is necessary to take precautions before legal incapacity occurs. Family caregivers' legal questions and concerns often entail the following issues (also see Questions 1):
- Legal capacity and capacity to testify, e.g., "Who certifies legal capacity?"
- Driving and capacity to drive, e.g., "Can my husband still drive a car despite suffering from dementia?" "What are the consequences of a car accident?"
- Power of attorney, e.g., "What does a power of attorney look like?" "Do I have to go to the notary for the power of attorney?"
- Legal support, e.g., "What is that?" "What are the consequences of legal support?"
- Living will, e.g., "Do I need a living will?"
- Accidents, e.g., "Who is liable for the damage?"

Questions 1. From family caregivers about legal aspects

- Why do I need a power of attorney at all?
- What is meant by guardianship? Is my family member then placed under disability?
- My family member refuses to talk to me about these things. They reject everything. What can I do?

Some issues can be dealt with by using problem-solving techniques in the therapy process (see Chapters 9 and 11). In most cases, however, it makes sense to refer to other specific counseling centers or regional Alzheimer's societies.

Case Examples 1 and 2 show typical concerns.

Conflicts cannot always be resolved as easily as they were in these two examples. It is, therefore, important for the family caregivers to obtain comprehensive information on legal issues. Various counseling centers and regional Alzheimer's societies can provide support in this regard (personal and telephone service).

3.5 Financial Questions

Caregiving and support tasks usually result in financial questions on the following topics:
- Care services, e.g., "How much money do the care services cost?"
- Semi-residential care, e.g., "How much does day care cost per day?" "Who bears the costs?"

Case Example 1. Dealing with finances

Ms. S. (70 years old) lives alone. Her daughter visits her daily and takes care of her mother living with dementia. Recently, it has happened more frequently that Ms. S. withdraws sums of money from her bank account that can no longer be found. Now Ms. S. has accused the neighbor of theft. The daughter then informs the surrounding neighbors about her mother's dementia and the resulting changes. This resolves the conflict with the neighbor. In addition, the daughter finds out about power of attorney for banks as well as for legal and financial issues, and she now makes sure that her mother always has enough money in "small bills" in her apartment for shopping.

Case Example 2. Driving a car

Mr. N. (69 years old) continued to drive his car despite his dementia. His wife was very concerned about this and feared that he might cause an accident. He himself showed no insight into the problem behavior and under no circumstances wanted to give up driving. For a while, Ms. N. always tried to be there when he drove, but this did not solve the problem. Together with her daughter, she was able to convince Mr. N. to give the car to their daughter, as she urgently needed the car for work. With a heavy heart Mr. N. gave the car to his daughter.

- Home expenses, e.g., "How much does a place in a nursing home cost?" "Who bears the cost?"
- Aids, e.g., "How much do the aids cost?" "Who bears the costs?"

It is not the aim of the therapy sessions to provide advice on financial issues. However, the therapist can provide support in contacting counseling centers and various offices (e.g., social services) by providing contact persons and addresses.

4 Diagnostic Tools for Caregiving of People With Dementia

For both psychotherapeutic practice and the evaluation of the effectiveness of the psychotherapeutic support for family caregivers, it is important to assess the caregiving situation, the psychological and physical stress, as well as the utilization of support. Measurements of the behavioral problems of the person with dementia that are assessed by the family caregivers can also provide important information and provide an insight into the difficulties of living together.

Should the family caregivers suffer from severe cognitive impairments themselves, psychotherapeutic treatment may be contraindicated. In this case, other support offers should be arranged as needed. In the case of people with dementia, dementia diagnostics should be suggested and carried out, if this has not already occurred.

The questionnaires presented in this chapter are based on experience from the intervention studies of my research group with family caregivers and on the recommendations by Moniz-Cook et al. (2008).

4.1 Questionnaires for Family Caregivers

4.1.1 Psychological and Physical Burden Measurements

As already explained in Chapter 1, family caregivers of people with dementia are confronted with extremely burdensome demands and life changes that can impair their health and quality of life. Since developing depressive symptoms is particularly common, it is recommended to use a measurement to assess depression. For this target group, the Center for Epidemiologic Studies Depression scale (Radloff, 1977) and the Hospital Anxiety and Depression Scale (Zigmond & Snaith, 1983) have been proven to be appropriate. Using these instruments, an initial assessment of clinically relevant depressive symptoms and subclinical symptoms can be made. In the case of clinically relevant symptoms, diagnostic clarification and sufficient long-term (if needed) psychotherapy treatment should always be recommended

Moreover, questionnaires on quality of life, caregiving burden, and physical health can provide important information and be used for evaluation. Box 2 provides an overview of assessments in these areas.

Box 2. Overview of questionnaires on family caregiver burden

Depressive symptoms and anxiety
• Center for Epidemiologic Studies Depression scale – CES-D (Radloff, 1977) • Hospital Anxiety and Depression Scale – HADS (Zigmond & Snaith, 1983)
Quality of life
• WHO Quality of Life assessment – WHOQOL-BREF (The WHOQOL Group, 1998)
Caregiver burden
• Short Sense of Competence Questionnaire – SSCQ (Vernooij-Dassen et al., 1999) • Zarit Burden Interview – ZBI (Zarit et al., 1980)
Physical health
• The 36-Item Short-Form Health Survey – SF-36 (Ware & Sherbourne, 1992)

4.1.2 Measurements of Specific Caregiving Situation Issues

In addition to the instruments listed in Box 2, other questionnaires can also be used for specific topics (summarized in Box 3). Although family caregivers are exposed to a lot of stress, not everyone perceives the caregiving situation as equally stressful, and many also report positive experiences in caregiving. The positive aspects of caregiving can be assessed with the Positive Aspects of Caregiving Questionnaire (Tarlow et al., 2004). The questionnaire consists of nine items that are assigned to the dimensions of self-affirmation (e.g., "Providing help to ... has made me feel good about myself") and outlook on life (e.g., "Providing help to ... has enabled me to appreciate life more").

Whether caregiving is appraised as burdensome or manageable depends on the caregiver's appraisal as to whether their available resources are sufficient to cope with the stressors. The Psychosocial Resource Utilization Questionnaire for Family Caregivers of People with Dementia measures the resource realization of family caregivers for people with dementia with a total of 36 items comprising three scales, Realization of Resources for Well-Being (nine items), Realization of Resources for Coping With Everyday Stress (20 items), and Realization of Resources for Social Support (seven items, Töpfer & Wilz, 2018).

Furthermore, dysfunctional thoughts and attitudes toward caregiving can contribute to and exacerbate stress and depressive symptoms. The Caregiver's Attitude Scale (Risch et al., 2022) measures dysfunctional as well as functional attitudes of the caregivers. The 28-item scale assesses caregiving thoughts in four distinct domains: dysfunctional caregiving standards, self-care, dysfunctional assumptions about dementia, and acceptance.

As described in Chapter 1, the loss of abilities and changes in personality caused by the disease can trigger the experience of grief. The Marwit-Meuser Caregiver Grief Inventory (Marwit & Meuser, 2002) was developed to measure caregiving-related grief (50 items divided into three factors). Personal Sacrifice and Burden measures what family caregivers have had to give up and the extent to which they experience personal loss. Heartfelt Sadness and Longing represents the emotional reaction, such as sadness toward the loss of the relationship with the care recipient. Worry and Felt Isolation refers to the extent to which family caregivers perceive the loss of personal relationships with others as a result of caregiving responsibilities and their concerns for the future.

The Caregiver Grief Scale by Meichsner et al. (2016) specifically assesses caregiving-related grief and includes items related to the avoidance of grief and its expression. This is important because some family caregivers avoid expressing their grief openly (e.g., crying or talking about it), due to a desire not to burden the person in need of care, or due to fear that expressing these feelings could lead to depression (Meichsner et al., 2016). The Caregiver Grief Scale comprises a total of 12 items assigned to four factors: Emotional Pain reflects the experience of grief and other painful emotions associated with the loss of a family member or loved one. The Relational Loss factor includes losses related to the relationship and what was shared with the care recipient when they were healthy, such as communication and daily activities. Absolute Loss refers to the absolute loss of the care recipient, the expectation of a future without that person, and the loss of meaning in life and the resulting despair. Acceptance of Loss measures both acceptance of dementia and grief response, including overt expression of grief.

The Texas Revised Inventory of Grief (Faschingbauer et al., 1987) refers to the time after a person's death.

As a reaction to being overwhelmed, a lack of support, as well as to other factors, family caregivers may also engage in verbal or physical violence in caregiving. The risk of abuse by family caregivers can be measured, for example, with the Caregiver Abuse Screen (Reis & Nahmiash, 1995). The tool consists of eight questions with binary answers to assess physical and psychological abuse and neglect. With the Modified Conflict Tactics Scale (Beach et al., 2005), family caregivers are asked how often they have acted psychologically and physically abusively toward the care recipient in the last 3 months, and provide their answers using a Likert-scale from 0 = *never* to 4 = *constantly*, with a value of ≥2 (sometimes) for each question indicating mistreatment. Five indicators of psychological abuse (screaming or shouting at the care recipient, threatening to send them to a nursing home, threatening to use physical violence, threatening to abandon them, and verbal abuse, e.g., using a harsh voice, insulting, swearing at, or calling them names), and five indicators of physical abuse (withholding food, hitting or slapping them, shaking them, handling them roughly in other ways, and whether the caregivers are afraid that they might hit or hurt the care recipient) are assessed.

Box 3. Overview of questionnaires on specific caregivers' issues

Positive aspects of caregiving and realization of psychosocial resources
• Positive Aspects of Caregiving Questionnaire – PACQ (Tarlow et al., 2004) • Psychosocial Resource Utilization Questionnaire for Family Caregivers of People with Dementia – PRUQ (Töpfer & Wilz, 2018)
Dysfunctional thoughts in caregiving
Caregiver's Attitude Scale – CAS (Risch et al., 2022)
Experience of grief and loss
• Caregiver Grief Scale – CGS (Meichsner et al., 2016) • Marwit-Meuser Caregiver Grief Inventory – MM-CGI (Marwit & Meuser, 2002) • Texas Revised Inventory of Grief – TRIG (Faschingbauer et al., 1987)
Verbal and latent violence in caregiving
• Caregiver Abuse Screen – CASE (Reis & Nahmiash, 1995) • Modified Conflict Tactics Scale – MCTS (Beach et al., 2005)

4.2 Questionnaires for the Subjective Assessment of Behavioral Problems in Dementia Patients

One instrument to assess the progression and severity of behavioral problems in dementia and the resulting experience of burden in family caregivers is the Behavioral Pathology in Alzheimer's Disease Rating Scale (Reisberg et al., 1987; Reisberg et al., 2014; Sittler et al., 2020).

Twenty-five characteristic behavior-related symptoms are asked about in a clinical interview with family caregivers or professional nurses. The following areas are inquired about: paranoid ideas or delusions, hallucinations, motor disorders, aggressiveness, circadian rhythm, affect disorders, fears, and phobia. The sum of the item ratings with a category yields the severity. The sum score for all categories represents the overall extent of the change in behavior, and a four-point global scale indicates the extent of the burden for the family caregivers.

4.3 Assessment of the Severity of Dementia

The Global Deterioration Scale (GDS, Reisberg et al., 1988) can be used to assess the severity of dementia. The different levels are distinguished by descriptions of the cognitive and functional deficits. An overview of the classification of the levels is presented in Box 4.

Box 4. Classification of the levels of the GDS (according to Reisberg et al., 1988)

Classification of Levels 1–7 of the GDS
Level 1: No cognitive decline
Level 2: Very mild cognitive decline
Level 3: Mild cognitive decline
Level 4: Moderate cognitive decline
Level 5: Moderately severe cognitive decline
Level 6: Severe cognitive decline
Level 7: Very severe cognitive decline

At the same time, the levels can be used to make a clinical assessment (normal – mild – moderate – severe) of the severity of the disease.

5
Therapist Attitude and Relationship Building

The recommendations in this chapter provide helpful information based on experience with family caregivers.

Rogers' (1951) three core conditions can be considered as the most important basis for building a relationship with family caregivers: positive regard, empathy, and congruence. They are particularly emphasized here, as recognition, appreciation, and empathy regarding the caregiving situation constitute the most important foundation for forming and maintaining a working alliance with the family caregivers. Most family caregivers are often there for the person with dementia around the clock and their well-being is thus under immense stress. What they are often missing is an appropriate recognition and/or understanding of their efforts. Thus, throughout the entire therapy process, the therapist should authentically and personally emphasize their appreciation and respect for the tremendous amount of effort that the family caregiver puts into caregiving.

Furthermore, from our experience, techniques for building a complementary relationship have proven to be particularly helpful (see Box 5).

For example, according to Sachse (2006, p. 2), a family caregiver with the interactive plan, "show yourself as competent," will behave in therapy in such a manner that they try very hard to show themself to the therapist as competent (e.g., by reporting what they are able to manage in caregiving while not mentioning the areas in which they have difficulties). By doing this, the family caregiver tries to receive the therapist's approval. Complementary behavior on the part of the therapists means recognizing the family caregiver as competent and signaling to them:
- I, the therapist, unquestionably recognize your competence in caregiving.
- I show you appreciation and recognition.
- You do not have to fight for it.
- You get everything you need here.

In doing so, the idea is that the therapist fulfills the caregiver's need for recognition, and the caregiver receives what they need in their relationship with the therapist. Thus, the caregiver obtains satisfaction and can therefore reduce their dysfunctional behavior (the desire to do everything *even better* with respect to caregiving). These positive experiences can then change dysfunctional schemas, from less perfectionism toward more self-care.

Box 5. Complementary relationship building (according to Sachse, 2006)

> "Complementary relationship-building means adapting the relationship-building to a very specific client. The therapist reconstructs relevant characteristics of a specific client and then aligns his/her relationship-building accordingly" (translated from German, Sachse, 2006, p. 34).
>
> Complementary behavior toward the client according to Sachse (2006, p. 73) means, also by using nonverbal signals, the following:
> - Show that one is interested in the person and the subject matter.
> - Signal that one is listening very attentively to the client and finds that what they say is relevant.
> - Signal that one takes everything the client says very seriously and gives thought to it.
> - Signal that one makes a great effort to understand and empathically comprehend the client and what they say.
>
> One should only do this if it can be done authentically. It is helpful to realize that the client also demands attention and respect and that it is okay to give them more of this if they need it to a greater extent.

5.1 The Caregivers Are Caregiving Experts

Example 1. Caregivers' impression regarding explantations about dementia and caregiving

> *Caregiver:* Yes, there are many books with reports about this disease that I have read. However, I got angry about how these things are sugarcoated. ... Well, I have the feeling that they all are saints that are taking care of the sick ... and everything that is difficult is only mentioned in passing. And sometimes I get angry about that.

The therapist should view the caregivers in principle as experts in their situation (see Examples 1 and 2). The caregivers have known their family member with dementia for many years and therefore know their "typical" behaviors (which may have also existed previously) and how to deal with them. This should always be validated and reinforced.

Additionally, caregivers can learn from their previous experience, including what they have learned in therapy, and reflect on which strategies have helped deal with the family member with dementia and which have led to conflicts. Here, the therapist can incorporate their experiences in the sense of: "Other family caregivers have told me that doing ... works well in everyday life. Maybe that would also be something that would be suitable for you. What do you think?" This demonstrates to family caregivers that they are the "caregiving experts," as they have intensive daily experiences with the person with dementia and have often already developed very creative ways of dealing with the person with dementia's changed behavior, which can also be useful for other family caregivers.

Example 2. Caregivers are the experts

> *Therapist:* Exactly. You are an expert in problem solving. We have already established that. That is something that ... Yes, that makes you, I think, a role model for other family caregivers as well ... how you find flexible solutions to deal with your husband, for example ... even though it's not very traditional or common ... that you ... that you sleep separately, because you realize that that is better for both of you.

When imparting psychoeducational content, therapists should not instruct or try to convince the caregivers. Thus, the focus should be on the caregiver's individual experiences in dealing with the person with dementia.

5.2 Normalizing and Depathologizing Counseling

Family caregivers often inadvertently get into care situations in which they experience stressful feelings and negative thoughts. Such experiences are normal and understandable given the challenging and highly stressful caregiving situation. Sessions with a psychologist or psychotherapist can, however, trigger feelings of insecurity and insufficiency in caregivers ("Because I fail at taking care of my husband, I have to see a therapist."). In order to prevent such an experience, the therapist should avoid assuming a higher ranking, expert position. A professional, compassionate, and caring attitude that conveys equality in the sense of, "What you experience is completely normal in your situation, it would be the same for me" is an important prerequisite for a supportive therapeutic relationship. It has also been shown to be beneficial if the therapist speaks about "our" feelings, "our" thoughts, and "our" reactions instead of giving the impression that only the caregivers feel and think a certain way (based on Eifert, 2011).

Case Example 3 illustrates family caregivers' barriers with respect to utilizing psychotherapeutic support. The accepting and encouraging attitude of the therapist in the session makes it easier for the family caregiver to express their concerns, fears, and also feelings of shame regarding the utilization of therapeutic support.

5.3 Family Caregivers Are Doing Their Best: Appreciation and Validation of Their Efforts

Example 3. Caregivers feel a lack of appreciation

> *Caregiver:* You are the suitor everywhere, you have to get down on your knees. It is the same when you say something somewhere as a family caregiver. I mean, I have the experience with *my* sick mother. It is not appreciated anywhere. You are the idiot *everywhere*, you are not appreciated at all.

As the statement in Example 3 made by the family caregiver shows, many of them want recognition and appreciation. Caregiving family members usually work very hard and sacrifice themselves for the well-being of the

Case Example 3. Barriers about utilizing psychotherapeutic support

The following excerpt stems from therapy with a 77-year-old caregiving wife.

Therapist: Great, I see that this is very important for you. You are really reflecting on that and are being very open.

Caregiver: Yes, I also have to say that I really spent time thinking about our sessions and I also read through the folder a few times. I also have the impression that I'm ready to want it too. Now that I have the help, I have to be open and honest, because there is no point in sugarcoating things with you.

Therapist: Yes.

Caregiver: Then we could stop the whole thing right away. Because then I wouldn't get anywhere.

Therapist: Yes. And I think that's great that you're ready now, it also takes courage.

Caregiver: Yes.

Therapist: And I think it's good that you are doing this for yourself.

Caregiver: When I was reflecting on our last session, I realized that I had said, admitted, and expressed things to you that I had never said to anyone before.

Therapist: Mm-hmm.

Caregiver: But that is also a matter of will.

Therapist: Yes.

Caregiver: I signed up also because I said to myself: "I certainly won't go into psychotherapy." But here, I can get an idea of how I can get help.

Therapist: Yes, great.

Caregiver: That would also be something that I would consider to be a goal.

Therapist: Yes, what we have just formulated: really accepting help and opening up a little.

Caregiver: Yes.

Therapist: Do you already have specific ideas for this, do you already have something in mind?

---

person with dementia. Throughout the entire therapy process, the therapist should therefore authentically and personally emphasize their appreciation and respect for the caregivers' tremendous efforts. Moreover, providing appreciation and recognition for the caregivers' efforts promotes their self-confidence and self-esteem (see Example 4).

Example 4. Valuation of the caregiver

Therapist: Where do you get all the energy for caregiving?

Caregiver: Yes, I actually ask myself that too.

Therapist: I find it really admirable how much effort you put forth.

However, the therapist can also get into a situation in which they cannot always immediately recognize and appreciate the caregivers' efforts, for example, when caregivers grumble about the family member with dementia or repeatedly and severely complain about difficulties in dealing with nurses, administrative bodies, or laws. The caregivers' experience of "No one sees all that I do" or "No one sees how hard I have it" is often concealed behind this. In these cases, family caregivers can usually only then be motivated to analyze actively, cope with, and change existing and future problems if they feel that they are perceived and understood by the therapist. Thus, caregivers experiencing this appreciation represents the prerequisite for building up a motivation to change. These family caregivers will only then be ready to pursue their own needs intensely if they have the feeling that the enormous effort they put forth every day is perceived and valued from the "outside" – in this case, from the therapist's side.

Moreover, some caregiving children hope to receive the longed-for recognition that has been absent throughout their whole life. Because the person with dementia is mostly not able to provide recognition, it is expected from other family members, especially from siblings, but also from friends and acquaintances. Such expectations may lead to conflicts and misunderstandings. In this context, therapy can provide a corrective framework in which family caregivers receive the missing recognition, which then leads to their ability to change. In the excerpt in Case Example 4, the therapist shows appreciation for the care provided and, at the same time, directly encourages the family caregiver to reinforce themselves, independent from others.

5.4 Isolation and Severe Suffering: Empathy and Patience

Family caregivers often have barriers to asking for, utilizing, and accepting support. This not only applies to caregiving but also areas of self-care. It is not uncommon for family caregivers to have no one with whom they can share and discuss the stressors of everyday life. Sometimes dysfunctional assumptions hinder the utilization of support. However, even friends and family often react with little interest or are overwhelmed by hearing the same problems repeatedly and being confronted with situations that can only be changed slightly or not at all. Thus, for many family caregivers, the therapy setting is the only framework in which they can discuss their problems and challenges in dealing with the person suffering from dementia (see Case Example 5). This requires the

---

Case Example 4. Encouraging the caregiver's self-reinforcement

The following excerpt stems from therapy with a 37-year-old caregiving daughter.

Therapist: Mm-hmm, you know what I notice? You are very good at praising others and are so hard on yourself.

Caregiver: Well, I'm not that hard on myself …

Therapist: Harder.

Caregiver: Yes, harder.

Therapist: And when I say, "I think you're doing it great. It's *really* okay how you're doing it," you then say, "Well, I don't believe that yet."

Caregiver: No, I'm not that convinced yet. I mean, if I had *completely* internalized that, I wouldn't have any problem at all. If I would think it's completely okay. I'm getting there slowly. … My father, a businessman, he never wanted to know much about problems, he was always exhausted anyway, tired. For him problems were way too much for him anyway, way too much, way too much. … and now with this dementia disease … Dad needs to be protected again, dad needs help again. And to realize that now and to say to myself: "So, you've done everything now, it's totally okay."

Case Example 5. Providing space for expressing burden

The following excerpt stems from therapy with a 59-year-old caregiving daughter.

Caregiver: Yes, that's okay with me. I always say to myself: I am not accountable to you. I can say what I think. I don't need to be afraid, I can express my thoughts and feelings, and that is important.

Therapist: Exactly, and I would like to reassure you about that. How much you are doing, and how much you have already done over the years is an incredible amount. And often outsiders cannot understand what is happening, they take it for granted, but it is not. This is a huge burden emotionally and physically.

Caregiver: Especially mentally. The emotional burden is much worse than the physical burden. They say: "Then get someone to wash her in the morning!" And so on. Then I say: "That's not it, that's not the burden." "To wash someone and dress them, that's not the worst. The mental stress is much, much worse."

therapist to take on a particularly patient approach. The experience has shown that it is useful to give the caregivers space at the beginning of each session to report on changes in everyday caregiving or their current situation. This provides an opportunity for the caregivers to experience some relief. Afterward, the therapy goals that were agreed upon can be worked on.

5.5 Unchangeable Burdens and Loss of Control: Confrontation and Acceptance

Family caregivers are confronted with a lot of unchangeable suffering, such as constant changes and losses (loss of the person with dementia's personality, loss of relationship and intimacy, etc.), as well as varying stressors (problem behaviors of the person with dementia, emergency situations, etc.). In view of this situation, our experience shows that it is particularly important for the therapist to internalize that this suffering can only be changed to a limited extent or not at all.

Therapists sometimes start to adopt a problem-solving perspective with the desire to change the situation in order to achieve a more bearable state for the family caregivers. This perspective is appropriate for single problems (searching for support services, changing behavior toward the person with dementia), but the suffering caused by dementia cannot be changed. Through an unsuitable, solution-oriented approach, the therapist can hinder constructive psychological processing. Thus, searching for solutions to situations that cannot be changed hinders the process of encouraging the acceptance of negative thoughts and feelings (emotion regulation processes), and, therefore, may maintain avoidance.

The sadness that caregivers experience in relation to the person with dementia's lack of ability to remember past situations cannot be reduced, for example, by training their cognitive abilities. The focus here is on accepting and allowing these feelings to exist. Coming to terms with negative emotions and the fact that many situations cannot be changed is consequently an important prerequisite for adapting to the changed situation. Many family caregivers are always searching for possible treatments for dementia themselves, for example, by following current studies on the cure for dementia, asking doctors to prescribe a new medication, doing cognitive exercises with the family member with dementia on a daily basis, or attributing changes in the family member with dementia to external circumstances, such as the weather, as illustrated in the Case Example 6 excerpt.

By adopting a more accepting attitude, the family caregivers can better manage to turn to the positive aspects of life again, and their preoccupation with the negative

---

Case Example 6. Lack of acceptance of the illness

The following excerpt stems from therapy with a 79-year-old caregiving wife.

Caregiver: Well, I think it's due to the weather now. He was much better in winter. As he is now, I can't understand him at all. He does weird things, and I think it's because of the sun. It's so warm now, and that's why he's like that.

Therapist: The thought is there that his changed behavior has something to do with the weather, right?

Caregiver: Yes, that's what I think.

Therapist: Could it be that behind that thought, there is also a bit of hope that it will get better again?

Caregiver: Yes, I think to myself, maybe ... yes! That I think: "Yes, if the weather changes again, then ..." Don't you think that it will then ...? Well, I hope that it will be better when it rains again and it's cooler.

Therapist: So, the hope that you're having is very understandable, and I can imagine well how you must feel. And very many caregivers find it very difficult to accept the course of the disease. This is something you obviously don't want. There is still hope that it will stagnate, or not go further down, or not get worse.

Caregiver: Yes.

Therapist: And I can just imagine that behind this thought, that it may be due to the weather, there is also a bit of hope: "Yes, if it is the weather, then it will change again!"

Caregiver: Yes.

Therapist: And then maybe it will get better again?

Caregiver: Now that the weather has become so beautiful, he has become more forgetful – in every way! Now he hardly recognizes his daughter anymore when she is with us. He asks me: "Yes, who is that sitting there?" So, he forgets things a lot and is not able to recognize people.

Therapist: Mm-hmm.

Caregiver: It's so strong now. You don't think it will stay that way now, do you?

Therapist: [Pauses] I don't think that can be excluded. I am very sorry to have to tell you.

Caregiver: Mm-hmm [disappointed].

Therapist: And, of course, I could tell you now, "Yes, it's the weather," and you might feel better about it, but …

Caregiver: No, no … you're right [aggrieved, starts to cry]. I have to face it … only then can I treat him appropriately.

Therapist: Yes. And that makes you very sad now …

Caregiver: Yes, but … I'm very glad you told me now.

changes caused by dementia can temporarily fade into the background. Acceptance can enable them to regain new energy and make changes in their lives, such as going to an event alone, although they were otherwise always accompanied by their (now ill) partner.

In summary, it is of particular importance that the therapist internalizes an attitude of acceptance themselves in order to be able to help the family caregivers with building acceptance.

6 Therapy Topics, Intervention Methods, and Framework

This chapter provides an overview of the topics, intervention methods, and framework of the Tele.TAnDem program as well as basic implementation guidelines.

In principle, specific topics and the appropriate interventions are determined individually for the family caregivers based on the respective problems, problem analyses, and goals and do not follow a fixed order. Instructions for therapists for the specific topics are presented in detail in Chapters 7–15. In general, a sound knowledge of dementia-specific issues is an essential prerequisite for delivering the therapy. Imparting dementia-specific knowledge is not part of this manual and is discussed only as an overview in Chapter 3.

An overview of the topics and corresponding interventions is provided in Table 2.

6.1 Individualized Therapy

Since dementia leads to very different demands and burden for the families concerned, a therapy tailored to the

Table 2. Topics and interventions

Topic	Intervention
First session and relationship building: Chapter 7	Shaping the first session and relationship building, exploring the problems, and determining the therapy goals.
Changing dysfunctional appraisals and thoughts: Chapter 8	Identifying and changing dysfunctional thoughts that aggravate caregiving.
Dealing with challenging behaviors: Chapter 9	Support for understanding and dealing with challenging behaviors.
Stress management and emotion regulation: Chapter 10	Imparting coping strategies for acute and burdening emotions such as anger and fury.
Self-care and scheduling pleasant and value-based activities: Chapter 11	Encouraging self-care and well-being.
Dealing with change, loss, and grief: Chapter 12	Assisting with processing and acceptance regarding changes, grief, and loss. Support in dealing with the redefinition of roles. Preparation for the death of the person with dementia.
Encouraging the utilization of informal and professional support: Chapter 13	Removing barriers to utilization, supporting caregivers in the search for and organization of professional help.
Limits to caregiving at home: Chapter 14	Support with respect to identifying the individual stress limit, decision making, planning and organization of institutional care.
Final session: Chapter 15	Shaping the final session and further recommendations.

individual needs and problems of the family caregivers is necessary. At the beginning of therapy, the specific life situation with respect to dementia and caregiving is explored in detail (see Chapter 7). Moreover, the individual caregiver's illnesses or other familial stress factors are also examined.

In view of the individual problems, caregiving and living situations, as well as the personality of the caregivers, it is decided in each case which intervention approaches and therapeutic strategies are necessary and helpful. For example, when working on the utilization of support services, it is crucial whether the caregivers have psychological or informational barriers. Accordingly, cognitive techniques are used to break down psychological barriers, such as changing specific dysfunctional thoughts ("I have to master the care alone"). In the case of information deficits, knowledge about financial and professional services is imparted.

6.2 Setting

The Tele.TAnDem program can be delivered via telephone as well as in person. It is usually much easier for family caregivers to receive the program via telephone or video, as it allows the caregivers' needs regarding time and place to be met. Moreover, delivery via remote therapy is advantageous if the family caregivers are ill themselves, are less mobile, or have no one to fill in for the caregiving duties while they are away. Telephone sessions prove to be particularly helpful for family caregivers in rural regions. Additionally, due to the more "anonymous" setting on the telephone, many caregivers can build trust more quickly and find it easier to talk about difficult topics. Other caregivers prefer face-to-face sessions if they are organizationally feasible.

The decision for the setting should above all be based on the needs of the caregivers, but also on the framework conditions in order to be able to offer the most effective support possible. In a face-to-face setting, the feasibility of adhering to the agreed appointments should be discussed with the caregivers, taking into consideration the journey, the organizational effort, and ensuring that the person with dementia is cared for.

If the therapy sessions take place over the phone, it should be discussed with the caregivers whether and how they can speak undisturbed. It should be ensured that the person with dementia cannot overhear or is not in the same room. However, disturbances are sometimes unavoidable. In this case, the family caregivers should be offered to continue the conversation at a later point in time.

6.3 Therapy Process and Structure of the Sessions

The therapeutic sessions can be divided into five phases (see Box 6). The intervention strategies can be selected, adapted, and then implemented based on Phase 1 (first session and relationship building) and Phase 2 (goal definition). However, in the process, it is often necessary to return to the initial phases, for example in order to consider new problems that may have arisen in the caregiving situation or that have been mentioned for the first time at a later point. It is important then to adapt the objectives accordingly, as the excerpt in Example 5 illustrates. Here the therapist provides support in reflecting on what has been achieved so far and in redefining goals.

Example 5. Interim evaluation and promotion of goal setting in the therapy process

> *Therapist:* I think it would be good if you again think about what you have found helpful in the sessions so far, what may have not been so helpful, and what you imagine and expect for the coming sessions. What you might need.

This recursive procedure enables an individual adaptation of therapy to the changed needs of the family caregivers in the course of the therapy.

Box 6. The five phases of the therapy process

> Phase 1: Diagnostics/first session and relationship building.
>
> Phase 2: Comprehending the individual problem situation and defining therapy goals.
>
> Phase 3: Selecting and individually adapting the intervention strategies.
>
> Phase 4: Implementing the interventions, if necessary redefining goals.
>
> Phase 5: Result and goal evaluation as well as completion of therapy.

The first and last therapy sessions entail specific content and a formal process that is based on specific goals: getting to know each other, exploration, and relationship building in the first session, and summary and evaluation in the last session. The shaping of these sessions is described in detail in Chapters 7 and 15. The following procedure has been proven to be effective for setting up the rest of the sessions: At the beginning, caregivers are asked about their current state and changes since the last sessions. Then, topics that were discussed last time should be addressed as well as the homework or transfer exercises. Next – based on the therapy goals – topics for the current session should be defined. The therapist should then select suitable intervention strategies and work on the topics together with the caregivers. At the end of the session, transfer exercises that are linked to the current session are agreed upon.

Occasionally, certain situations may make it necessary to deviate from this structure, for example building a necessary complementary relationship with caregivers who are particularly burdened or who are experiencing particularly serious problems with caregiving, or if the person with dementia has been placed in a home or has died. Such crises always have priority over the topics that were initially planned for the respective session.

The following materials can be used while delivering the program:
1. Treatment manual for the therapists.
2. Worksheets for the family caregivers. In the case of telephone therapy, these are sent as a workbook including a photo of the therapist.
3. If necessary, brochures on certain topics (e.g., incontinence, local, and regional support services).

6.4 Work Between Sessions: Therapeutic Homework

The use of psychotherapeutic homework is usually important and helpful for the transfer of the topics learned in therapy to everyday life.

Appropriate cognitive behavioral interventions are implemented to help family caregivers cope with burdening situations when dealing with the persons with dementia (e.g., by applying certain behavioral strategies or cognitive restructuring). These interventions are used, for example, to schedule pleasant activities, to utilize social and/or professional support, or to cope with burdening emotions such as feelings of grief. Importantly, the interventions focus on the caregiving situation in everyday life and thus on the time between the therapy sessions (and/or the time after therapy completion). Thus, the use of therapeutic homework is of great importance. However, since the family caregivers are already heavily stressed in their everyday life and have severe time constraints, they should be given appropriate tasks that can be implemented in a timely manner in order to avoid additional stress. It is thus imperative when working with family caregivers to select homework wisely and make sure not to overtax them with additional homework or tasks. It is also helpful, especially for older family caregivers, to have a written reminder drawn up at the end of the session. Possible homework assignments are listed in Box 7.

Box 7. Therapeutic homework

Cognitive tasks
Observing/protocolizing (e.g., recognizing and writing down dysfunctional thoughts)
Preparing decisions (e.g., obtaining missing information, making phone calls)
Reflecting (e.g., thinking about self-care)
Psychoeducation/bibliotherapy (e.g., reading information about dementia)
Behavioral tasks
Confrontational tasks (e.g., going out in public with the person with dementia)
Changing behavior (e.g., changing how one deals with the person with dementia)
Mindfulness and self-care (e.g., practicing relaxation procedures daily, pursuing a hobby)
Creative tasks (e.g., writing a letter to oneself)
Interpersonal tasks (e.g., asking another person for help with caregiving, maintaining social contacts)
Behavioral experiments (e.g., checking one's own expectations)
Impulse control (e.g., emotion regulation exercise for dealing with anger)

7 First Session and Relationship Building

In the first session, the focus is on relationship building and clarifying the content and goals of the therapy sessions. Since family caregivers usually do not have any mental disorders, it is first important to create an understanding of what psychotherapeutic interventions look like in their specific case and what kind of support can be given. The motivation to participate is heterogeneous among family caregivers. It ranges from a clearly defined and formulated caregiving-related concern to digressions regarding the unbearable, stressful, and hopeless caregiving situation, for which no help seems possible.

Therefore, in this chapter, relationship building during the first contact, getting to know the caregiving situation, the analysis of the main problem areas, as well as goal definition are discussed.

7.1 Goals of the Module

In addition to the establishment of the therapeutic relationship, suggestions are given in particular to develop a motivation for change, since the motivation for change is not present in all family caregivers. Further focal points of the module are the analysis and selection of individual main problem areas in everyday caregiving as well as goal definition.

7.2 Therapeutic Approach

In this section, the therapeutic approach is discussed in more detail by introducing the various treatment methods that are listed in Box 8.

Box 8. Overview of the interventions

- Relationship building and imparting knowledge
- Exploring the caregiving situation
- Analysis and identification of the main problem areas
- Building motivation for change
- Defining goals
- Concluding the first session

7.2.1 Relationship Building and Imparting Knowledge

In principle, family caregivers are to be viewed as experts in their caregiving situation. This mindset, as well as esteem and appreciation with respect to the caregiving efforts, represent the central and fundamental characteristics of shaping the relationship. Depending on the caregiver's concerns and personality, different aspects could be important for shaping the therapeutic relationship. Examples of different forms of shaping the interaction in the initial therapy sessions, as well as in the preceding discussions, are presented in Chapter 5.

Another central aspect in the initial session is to provide space for family caregivers to find relief. It is important for the therapist to provide a high degree of individual care and attention to the caregiver in order to meet their needs in terms of the considerable amount of pressure they are under. The therapist should always acknowledge the client's responsibility to provide caregiving, their efforts, and their experience of burden. Since family caregivers often do not have an empathetic listener with whom they can speak about caregiving burden in detail, most family caregivers experience the therapist's recognition as very supportive and soothing.

Speaking in detail about the current situation can, however, also actualize the problem and thus can be very stirring and burdensome for the caregivers, as the excerpt in Example 6 illustrates.

Example 6. Problem actualization through the first session

> *Caregiver:* At the moment, I'm a little ... I don't know if the first talk with you stirred me up, but I've kind of been in a mess since then. Well, I don't know if it has anything to do with that, but I ruminate a little more now and am not sleeping as well; maybe something got triggered somehow.
>
> *Therapist:* Yes, so, you suspect that speaking to me about the various areas that are moving you at the moment triggered something again, so that you sleep a little worse, ruminate more. Right?
>
> *Caregiver:* Yes, exactly.
>
> *Therapist:* What are your main thoughts, or what is occupying you?

However, focusing on the problems is a necessary prerequisite in order to be able to analyze and work on them. Moreover, it also promotes emotional processing (see Chapters 10 and 12).

In addition to exploring the caregiving situation, it is essential to communicate information on the organization, topics, and goals of therapeutic support in the first session. The following aspects should be addressed:
- frequency, time structure, and duration of the sessions;
- planned or possible topics;
- planned therapeutic approaches;
- limits of therapeutic support;
- materials/handouts; and
- confidentiality.

Furthermore, it should be emphasized that a nuanced planning of the therapy sessions can only occur if adequate information about the caregiving situation and the person with dementia is provided.

7.2.2 Exploring the Caregiving Situation

Exploring the caregiving situation and the clinical picture of the person with dementia should be the focus in the first session in order to acquire a first impression of the existing requirements and burdens. Here, it is helpful when the caregiver describes their life together and/or the caregiving situation, as well as the resulting changes regarding their own health and quality of life. The best way to do this is to use an open, narrative questioning style that encourages the caregiver to talk about everyday caregiving and interactions with the person with dementia (see Example 7).

Example 7. Talking about everyday caregiving

> *Therapist:* Mrs. E., so that I can get a little bit of an impression, maybe tell me about a typical day in your life right now. What does that look like?

Some caregivers on the other hand expect a more active information-gathering role from the therapist and find it easier to answer specific questions. Questions 2 highlights questions that are suitable for this approach.

Questions 2. Explore the caregiving situation

- What kind of help do you give your family member?
- What does your help/caregiving look like in everyday life?
- How much time did you spend on average in the last week on helping/caring for your family member during the day/night?
- What is the maximum amount of time you can leave your family member at home alone without supervision?
- What burdens you the most about the caregiving situation?
- Has your health and quality of life changed since you started caregiving?

In the next step, the clinical picture and course of the syndrome can be explored. Here information can be obtained on the duration of the burden as well as specific problem areas related to the specific symptoms of dementia (Questions 3).

Questions 3. About dementia

- When did your family member show the first signs of dementia?
- How long ago was the medical diagnosis made?
- Since when has your family member been suffering from dementia?
- Do you know what type of dementia your family member has?
- What impairments does your family member have?

It is also important to explore the utilization of support services as well as the desire for further support. Among other things, this information provides a basis for the later planning of positive and value-based activities (Questions 4).

Questions 4. Exploration of the utilization of support services

- Is there someone who can look after your family member when you are away or sick?
- How difficult is it to find someone on an hourly basis?
- How difficult is it to find someone on a daily basis?
- Do you receive support in looking after/caring for your family member?
- Have you made use of any support services in the past 6 months?
- How many days per month do you use this support?
- Would you like more or different support?

In addition to exploring problem areas and burdens, it is very important to inquire about the caregivers' resources and coping strategies as well as the positive aspects of caregiving. Questions 5 can be used for this.

Questions 5. Resource-oriented questions regarding the caregiving situation

- Please imagine a normal week: What do you do for yourself to provide relief?
- How do you regain your strength?
- Even a stressful situation can have many sides: What positive aspects have you experienced in caregiving?

7.2.3 Analysis and Selection of the Main Problem Areas

By exploring the caregiving situation and the person with dementia's symptoms, family caregivers usually describe a large number of burdens and problems. Based on this, more differentiated inquires can be made regarding how the caregivers experience these specific situations as well as whether, and in what way, they would like to change something in these problem areas.

For understanding conflicts in nursing, behavioral analyses can be very helpful, which also provide important insights into stressful, dysfunctional thoughts and sustaining factors. The procedure for carrying out behavioral analyses is outlined in Chapter 9.

In the next step, caregivers are asked to assess and rank the discussed problem areas according to their subjective stress level. On the basis of this assessment (ranking list), the caregivers can select which problem areas should be dealt with in the therapy sessions. As a rule, no more than three main problems should be specified so that there is sufficient time to deal with them and find successful solutions (see Example 8). It may be necessary for the therapist to assist in selecting the problem areas with regard to whether they can be worked on in the therapy sessions.

Example 8. Starting the topic of analyzing and selecting main problem areas

> *Therapist:* In the sessions I would like to help you to find beneficial starting points for changes and relief. Therefore, it would be helpful if you told me how you experience caregiving and supporting your family member with dementia and what problem areas exist. We will then pick out one or two particularly stressful situations and you can try to describe to me in detail what exactly is difficult about it. Then I would like to know what you think would make your situation easier, what you wish for, or what you would like to change.

In individual cases, family caregivers may bring so many different problem areas into the therapy that, at first, there is no "common thread," and it is difficult to structure them into a few main problem areas that can be worked on. It may be that not just one person is being cared for, but several (e.g., the husband suffering from dementia and the mother), or that the caregivers still have a full-time job and provide care simultaneously. Especially caregiving daughters are frequently faced with the challenges of having to coordinate raising their own children with caregiving. Often, there are also financial problems and constraints that make it difficult to utilize external support services. In such cases, it is important first to work out priorities with the caregivers and to point out the limits of psychotherapeutic interventions. A caregiving daughter who simultaneously has a full-time job, has a small child at home, and is taking care of a parent is likely to be overwhelmed in the long term. In such cases, authentic feedback, combined with expressing one's own concern about the many tasks to be mastered, is an important psychotherapeutic method for developing motivation to change.

7.2.4 Developing Motivation to Change

For some family caregivers, the motivation to see a psychologist or participate in a psychotherapeutic program can be based on the desire to do something for the person with dementia. In these cases, self-care or dealing with one's own stress as a reason for participation are not mentioned initially: "I'm participating because of my family member who is ill. In order to be able to provide care for him even better." In such cases, it should first be discussed with the caregivers that this is not the primary goal of the psychotherapeutic sessions (see Example 9).

Example 9. Self-care

> *Therapist:* Taking care of yourself is just as important as taking care of your family member with dementia. Because caregiving for your ... is not possible in the long term if you're not in good health!

The condition of the person with dementia can also improve if the caregivers are accompanied and supported in dealing with the syndrome and its effects. It should therefore be emphasized to the caregivers that they themselves are the focus of the therapy, that the aim is to restore their well-being, and that they also have a right to attention, support, as well as their own needs outside of the caregiving situation. This focus on the caregivers should be emphasized by the therapist throughout the course of the therapy. It is easier for relatives to accept this point of view if, with the support of the therapist, they keep in mind that they can only guarantee long-term care if they take good care of themselves and use support services (see Case Example 7).

7.2.5 Goal Definition

Compared to psychotherapy patients, who are usually able to express their wishes more clearly ("I want to reduce my anxiety" or "I want to feel joy in life again"), caregivers do not always clearly formulate their goals. Many family caregivers sign up for therapeutic support and report severe stress but do not raise a specific issue they would like to work on. Especially in the first session, caregivers sometimes cannot state a specific concern that they would like to work on and/or cannot select one from the abundance of burdens. Altogether, it is important for the therapeutic process to provide sufficient time to discuss the burdens and describe the caregiving and living situation. It is thus possible that the analysis of the main problem areas and goal setting requires multiple therapy sessions to complete. Therefore, caregivers should not be rushed to find therapy goals.

In some cases, it is only the therapist who initially has a clear picture of which issues should be worked on, even if the caregivers are not aware of them at the time; for example, issues such as dealing with grief or encouraging acceptance of the illness. Therefore, the therapy sessions can be meaningful and helpful even without a jointly defined goal and can follow a therapeutic structure in terms of content (see Case Example 8). Generally, implicit problem processing and goals can be communicated well and openly at a later time point in therapy.

Experience also shows that the concern of some family caregivers, who cannot state specific goals but would still like to receive therapeutic support, is to receive recognition and appreciation for their effort in caregiving. This desire is understandable since many family caregivers do not receive recognition in their social environment. From our point of view, it can also be a therapeutic task to give

---

Case Example 7. Therapeutic work on motivation to change

The following excerpt stems from therapy with a 56-year-old caregiving daughter.

Therapist: Perhaps we can take a look together again to find out how you can be calmer. I would suggest to you, Mrs. M., that you work on the What Would I Like to Achieve? worksheet before our next session and see again whether there is anything you would like to change. You can take time on the questions and think about what exactly the change might look like; what your idea would be on how to get there.

Caregiver: Yes, you know, the problem is: to change something, is something active.

Therapist: Yes, that's right.

Caregiver: And I already struggle to manage everyday life.

Therapist: Could you still imagine taking a look at it again before our next session and think about it?

Caregiver: I've already been thinking about it for a long time, at least 7 or 8 years.

Therapist: Maybe it would be very helpful to approach it in a somewhat structured way.

Caregiver: Should I write something down?

Therapist: Yes, I think that would be great. Until next time.

this recognition and, at the same time, support family caregivers in building up self-esteem in order to make themselves more independent from others' feedback.

Some caregivers can already state specific goals in the first session that can be worked on within the therapeutic process. In the case of behavior-related goals, Goal Attainment Scaling (GAS, Kiresuk & Sherman, 1968) is suitable for specifying and evaluating them (see Worksheet 7-2 in the Appendix).

Questions 6 suggests questions that are helpful for specifying the goals.

Questions 6. Specifying the goals

- How important is a change for you?
- What would make the situation easier for you?
- What would make you feel better or less stressed?
- What are your own needs in the situation?

Possible obstacles to achieving the goals should also be considered. Questions 7 gives questions that are suitable for this.

Questions 7. Obstacles to achieving the goals

- What are you afraid of with respect to achieving your goals?
- Are the goals possibly conflicting with what your family/family members have in mind?
- What would the current situation be like if you had already achieved your goal?
- How do others see the problem?

Goal Attainment Scaling is, however, not suitable for all relevant goals. For example, processing losses and encouraging acceptance may not be definable on a numerical scale (Case Example 9).

7.2.6 Concluding the First Session

At the end of the first session, a short summary of the results of the session, the topics of the next session, as well as the date and time for the next session should be given. In addition, any open questions should be clarified. In principle, caregivers are encouraged to ask questions and to express expectations, anticipatory anxiety,

---

Case Example 8. Therapeutic work on finding goals

The following excerpt stems from therapy with a 75-year-old caregiving wife.

Caregiver: Basically, it helps me a lot when I can talk to someone. That's how it is here ... and it helps me.

Therapist: Yes, and then we can still work together so that we – in addition to you letting everything out that moves you – can take a more directed look and work out what you want to address in our sessions. What do you want to change?

Caregiver: Yes, that I don't get so upset about certain circumstances and situations. On the other hand, as I said, something is changing for me now. I feel kind of sad when nobody comes to visit me. Actually ... I'm slowly wanting only peace and quiet. I know that this is actually a harmful development, but there is also a certain amount of peace that comes with it, you know? But actually, from my nature –

Therapist: You know that you don't actually know this part of yourself?

Caregiver: Yes.

Therapist: Such exhaustion, such a tendency to withdrawal?

Case Example 9. Therapeutic work on defining goals

Therapist: Yes, okay. If you were to state what you want now: What should be changed so that you feel better?

Caregiver: Yes, basically I think that I am already realistic and stable, but I just have the impression that my mind is telling me something different than my feeling. And this feeling keeps constantly compelling me to go against it instead of accepting it.

Therapist: Yes. That is, you want more acceptance and emotional processing, so that you can distance yourself from it a bit.

Caregiver: Yes, that the mind gets a little more weight.

Therapist: Specifically, it is about the situation in which your wife reacts with accusations.

Caregiver: Yes, I wish to be more patient in certain situations and also to respond to her in an understanding manner … that I just wait longer and don't always dictate that things have to go this or that way … that when she goes for a walk, to just let her walk as she wants. That I don't look at the clock and think: "But she has to be back home in 2 hours. If we walk around there or there, we won't make it." Yes, I always disrupt her will, I would say, and I think that maybe that's why she gets annoyed and always looks at me again like, "What does he want again now?" That's the impression she gives me. I should just be a little more nonchalant.

Therapist: That would certainly be important to see what is happening in such situations: "How can I maybe deal with it differently? Where can I give her space? Where do I have to intervene?" But I also understand that you sometimes have to say: "So, now let's do this and that."

Caregiver: Yes.

Therapist: And it would also be important that you don't feel so guilty afterward.

Caregiver: That too, yes. When she looks at me like that sometimes, it hurts so much.

Therapist: Yes, yes.

Caregiver: Yes, and that I just … I don't know.

Therapist: Dealing with feelings of guilt, with conflicts in day-to-day caregiving, maybe?

Caregiver: Yes, that's exactly it.

Therapist: Yes, maybe we should write that goal down on the worksheet under goal one.

Caregiver: Yes.

Therapist: So, dealing with feelings of guilt and conflicts in day-to-day caregiving?

Caregiver: Yes, that would then probably provide some relief for everyday situations and help me be at peace with myself.

Therapist: When these feelings arise, you quickly get the feeling that you have done something wrong and that maybe you have to do it differently. Often such feelings are not proof that we actually did something wrong … it doesn't necessarily mean that you did something wrong.

Caregiver: Yes, that's exactly what I think. If someone comes over and experiences it for 2 hours, I always get the impression that they are trying to tell me: "You can't do it like this, you can't do it like that." They don't say that, but I always get the impression that they want to convey to me: "Don't be like that. You're doing too much, too little, or you're doing it wrong."

Therapist: And that's where you want more self-confidence.

Caregiver: Mm-hmm.

Therapist: I think this is a very important point with the feelings that arise in the various situations that something has been done wrong, although the person suffering from dementia behaves this way because of their own insecurity, because of the illness, and not because you actually did something wrong.

Caregiver: Yes, exactly.

Therapist: What would you wish for in dealing with these feelings, what would you like to achieve?

Caregiver: Actually, I would like to become a little more hard-nosed.

Therapist: Yes, so to get a little distance.

Caregiver: So, I think that, um, if it wasn't my wife, but my father or mother, um, that I could react differently.

and insecurities. Encouraging prompts are helpful for this, such as shown in Questions 8.

Questions 8. Encouraging prompts

- Do you have any questions about … (procedure, confidentiality, etc.)?
- Does what we've talked about so far meet your expectations? What are your expectations for the sessions/me?
- Is there anything that you have not yet understood?
- Are there any concerns on your part? Do you see any particular obstacles or difficulties related to our sessions?

Finally, the caregivers should be asked how they are doing at the moment, as detailed discussion of problems can be stressful. Resource-oriented inquiries about what would be good for the caregivers after the session can also divert the focus to self-care. Note that resource activation and self-care are important aspects that are continually pursued throughout the entire therapy process (Example 10).

Example 10. Exploration of caregiver's feelings

Therapist: How do you feel now?

Caregiver: Good. Grateful that I was able to tell you all about it.

8 "I Grew Up in the Countryside, and That Was a Given There": Changing Dysfunctional Thoughts and Appraisals

" ... and I noticed that he always needed more help, and well ... I'm his wife." "'In good times and in bad times' is what we said many, many years ago, and yes, now I am trying to realize that."

Caregiving and the associated stressful conditions are evaluated and experienced differently by different people. For some, care is a manageable task, while others suffer from the complex demands. Moreover, dysfunctional attitudes and appraisals regarding care increase the burden.

For many family members, taking on the responsibility of providing care is seen as a matter of course and is not reflected on. In this way, family care is classified as a necessary, unchangeable duty based on cultural, family, and personal values and norms. However, particularly for family members who are under a lot of burden, it can be very helpful to consciously reflect on and question the decision to take on caregiving.

Furthermore, excessive demands regarding the way in which care is to be carried out can exponentiate the requirements. For instance, many caregivers have perfectionistic standards regarding caregiving. This often coincides with nonutilization of professional support. Reasons for this are specific attitudes, for example that caregiving "must" be provided on one's own or that "strangers" cannot provide adequate help for the person with dementia. The use of support can also be seen as a personal failure, so some caregivers do not ask for help out of shame or difficulties with accepting help.

Dysfunctional thoughts can also cause very burdensome feelings of guilt. For instance, some family members blame themselves for the disease, because in the past they behaved negatively and stressfully toward the person with dementia, or they feel guilty and have a bad conscience if they subjectively do not perform caregiving well enough, temporarily hand it over to someone else, or pay attention to their own needs. Caregivers also often have stress-promoting appraisals of the person with dementia's behavior. Family members often experience the person with dementia's behavior as an expression of spite, ignorance, and defiance. This misinterpretation can lead to conflicts with the person with dementia and can be emotionally burdensome.

Box 9 provides an insight into stress-promoting/dysfunctional thoughts and attitudes that are often expressed by caregivers.

Box 9. Examples of caregivers' typical dysfunctional thoughts and attitudes

Sense of duty and perfectionism in caregiving

- I must always be available to my wife.
- I am solely responsible for the care.
- I only ask for help when I cannot do it anymore.
- I'm only doing well if he is well.
- I find it a disgrace to my husband when a nurse comes into the house.
- I am not allowed to make any mistakes during caregiving.
- Sometimes I think that I am a bad person because I cannot manage it any better.

Feelings of guilt

- Sometimes I think that I might be partly to blame for my loved one's dementia.
- If my loved one is not doing well, I blame myself.
- I am to blame if she no longer wants to eat. Maybe I did not care well enough.
- I feel bad about doing something good for myself when my loved one might need me.
- I could not endure the feelings of guilt, if I would place my mother in a home.

> **Misjudgments of personality changes and challenging behaviors**
>
> - My loved one could be more thankful that I am always there for him.
> - My family member deliberately makes life difficult for me.
> - My loved one is not really trying. When others are there, he tries.
> - He actually knows where everything is. He just wants to be served.
>
> **Feelings of shame and denial**
>
> - He makes a fool of both of us with his behavior.
> - I would be embarrassed if others saw him like that. Therefore, I do not want a visiting service.
> - No one should notice that he is ill.
> - In winter he is usually worse off. In spring it will certainly get better again when we can be outside in the garden. Until then, I can manage it alone.

The dysfunctional thoughts and attitudes described in Box 9 were identified as an essential predictor of the degree of experienced mental stress (Losada et al., 2010). Furthermore, dysfunctional thoughts are associated with increased depressive symptoms (McNaughton et al., 1995), which in turn can considerably curtail everyday functioning and the quality of interpersonal relationships. Dysfunctional thoughts thus additionally complicate the caregiving situation as well as a healthy balance between taking responsibility for the person with dementia and maintaining one's own mental and physical well-being. Therefore, changing these dysfunctional thoughts is an essential intervention goal, which can be worked toward by using cognitive restructuring techniques.

8.1 Goals of the Module

Through cognitive restructuring methods, family caregivers can learn to identify their often debilitating and discouraging thoughts and develop alternative, more helpful thoughts.

In addition, the effect of thoughts on emotions and experience of burden are explained to the family caregivers. The underlying assumption is that the appraisal of an event determines one's own emotional state. Together with the family caregivers, therapists illustrate that negative thoughts elicit reactions that lead to tension and burdensome feelings and that these feelings in turn cause certain behavior. Therefore, caregivers' inadequate, unhelpful assumptions are questioned, possibilities for changing them are discussed, and alternative thoughts and behavioral patterns are developed. The alternative thoughts and behavioral patterns developed by using Socratic dialogue and guided discovery should then progressively be established in the individual life situation (transfer).

This chapter focuses in particular on cognitive interventions to work on the sense of duty, personal/family norms, and perfectionism. Cognitive interventions to modify dysfunctional assumptions regarding the person with dementia's behavior (misinterpretation of personality changes and challenging behaviors as well as dealing with feelings of shame) are addressed in Chapter 9, cognitive interventions to promote self-care in Chapter 11, and the critical examination of feelings of guilt in Chapter 12. However, the therapeutic approach follows the same basic principles of cognitive restructuring for all of the problem areas mentioned in Box 9. Box 10 contains an overview of the interventions covered in this chapter.

Box 10. Overview of the interventions

> - Identification of dysfunctional thoughts, attitudes, and schemes
> - Critical examination of dysfunctional assumptions (Socratic dialogue) including imagery exercises
> - Development of alternative, helpful thoughts
> - Imparting the ABC model (Ellis, 1977)

8.2 Therapeutic Approach

8.2.1 Identifying, Challenging, and Criticial Examination of Dysfunctional Thoughts

Dysfunctional thoughts and attitudes are usually already evident in the initial consultation. However, the schemes and automatic thoughts, which are usually shaped biographically, are not perceived and addressed by the family caregivers as a problem. The therapist thus forms their own hypotheses about dysfunctional schemas and thoughts as well as the clients' backgrounds, triggers, and functionality (see Chapter 7). In the therapeutic process, the therapist increasingly uses open, and sometimes confrontational, questions to guide the family caregivers to perceive their dysfunctional thoughts and appraisals and to recognize inconsistencies themselves. Through guided discovery, alternative, helpful thoughts and appraisals are eventually developed. Therefore, specific questions, which are summarized in Table 3, could be useful.

Feelings of duty regarding taking over care are a typical and frequent topic in the therapeutic work with caregiving daughters and daughters-in-law (see also further literature by Geister, 2004, "Because I am responsible for my mother" [German: "Weil ich für meine Mutter verantwortlich bin."]). The questioning of these feelings of duty and personal values is always carried out with the aim of counteracting caregivers' overload and associated health impairments. However, the work on these norms and values should not be misunderstood as a direct exercise of influence on the caregivers' desire and decision to provide care at home and in a self-determined manner.

The excerpts in Case Examples 10, 11, and 12 illustrate the therapeutic process concerning the perception of, reflection on, and questioning of internalized norms regarding responsibility and duty of care.

Table 3. Helpful questions for cognitive restructuring

Helpful questions for cognitive restructuring	
Reality testing	• Do you remember experiences that showed that this thought is not always appropriate? • Which evidence/facts speak for/against your point of view? • Which other possibilities could explain the situation? • These are the negative aspects of the situation. Are there also positive aspects? • In your appraisal of the situation, do you take responsibility for things over which you have no control? • Are there perhaps small, easy-to-overlook details in the situation that would speak against your thoughts or lead to a different evaluation?
Mood-enhancing thoughts	• How do you feel when you have these thoughts? • Does the thought help you feel how you want to feel? • Does the thought help you cope well with the situation? • In a different emotional state, when you are doing well for example, do you then think differently about this situation? How?
Changing perspective	• What would you say to a good friend if they had this thought? • What would a good friend say to you in this situation if they knew about this thought and were not completely convinced regarding its accuracy? • Do you know someone who can cope with this situation more easily than you? What might this person say to themselves?
Changing perspective related to time	• How will you think about this in the future, in a month or in a year? • Imagine yourself 10 years later. How would you view the current situation looking back? From this perspective, is the focus on other aspects?
Decatastrophizing	• What is the worst thing that could happen? How bad would that really be? How likely is that? • What would be worse than this situation? • How important is this thing really for you?
Focus on resources and competence	• Have you ever mastered a similarly difficult situation? How did you manage it then? What helped you? • Is there something that is very important to you that you might remember in this situation and that can give you courage and inner security? • What can you trust in?
Search for meaning	• What can you learn in this situation? • What meaning do you find in caregiving?

In addition, the case examples show that the discussed values and attitudes have a biographical origin and in this context are comprehensible and workable. The identification and disputation of biographically anchored schemas require a longer communication process, so the case examples in this chapter are correspondingly extensive.

In Case Example 10, a caregiving daughter's taking on care is questioned, because she reports significant health impairments due to the multiple-stress situation caused by care, work, and her own family. The therapist disputes the internalized norms, illustrates the biographical background and the consequences, confronts the caregiving daughter with the lack of support from the family, and encourages a self-care-related point of view.

The next dialogue, Case Example 11 focuses on the processing of dysfunctional schemas regarding one's own responsibility for the well-being of the person with dementia. This case example will also illustrate that burdensome attitudes are based on biographical experiences and are viewed in this context. Accordingly, a longer section of the conversation was selected so that the gradual cognitive change process can be understood. However, this sequence represents only a small part of the whole disputation.

> **Case Example 10. Duty fulfillment and perfectionism**
>
> The following excerpt stems from therapy with a 56-year-old caregiving daughter.
>
> *Therapist:* So, what you are describing to me now is really serious. That you notice it physically, that you notice palpitations, that you are tense, that you are to some extent tearful, that you are irritated very quickly, and then there's your retired husband who's also at home, and who also wants your attention. ... Yes, that you notice that it's really exhausting. Probably always such a balancing act. To be at work and to know: "That's not something I can leave behind. The children want to be supported. I have to finish my job, it has to be done," while, on the other hand, knowing, that hopefully nothing happens to your father: "I also have to go home, he's not being looked after properly right now. He's not been moved. What is he eating?"
>
> *Caregiver:* Well, that's how we were raised, to do everything correctly. We were brought up to strive for perfection. Maybe that's why. For example, if we felt sick as children, they said, "You're going to school anyway."
>
> *Therapist:* So, to live up to the expectations of others, and not listen to the signals your body sends you?
>
> *Caregiver:* Yes.
>
> *Therapist:* That you ignore the signals of your mood and your body and instead look at what expectations and requirements of others you should meet. This seems to me to be a rather old pattern. This pattern, which is now getting to you, was certainly in your life before, but it has not pushed you to the limits as it is doing currently.
>
> *Caregiver:* Yes.
>
> *Therapist:* What are you avoiding here? That someone will reproach you? If you think it through to the end.
>
> *Caregiver:* No, no one would reproach me, because they all want me to lighten my load and give my father away. But perhaps I think subconsciously: "Ah yes, now you didn't take care of him until death. So many other people manage to do it, and you can't even manage that."
>
> *Therapist:* Hmm, so that's like a ...
>
> *Caregiver:* Like a compulsion.
>
> *Therapist:* So, an ideal that you've internalized: That you want or should care for your father at home until the end.
>
> *Caregiver:* Yes, mm-hmm.
>
> *Therapist:* Do you have an idea of where this firm belief, to care for your father at home until the end, comes from?
>
> *Caregiver:* Maybe this was set as an example for me, when my grandpa was being cared for. That was a given in my environment. I was raised in the countryside and that was a given there.

Therapist: And what were the conditions under which your grandpa was cared for?

Caregiver: Well of course they had it easier, because the whole family also lived nearby.

Therapist: Mm-hmm, okay. So, there were also other relatives there. How many people split up the care?

Caregiver: Yes, well, they all lived nearby; four of them split up the care.

Therapist: Okay. So, four family members split up the care. And how is your situation?

Caregiver: I'm by myself.

Therapist: You're by yourself. And completely, aren't you? So, your husband, he is nice and sweet, but he barely supports you, correct?

Caregiver: No, not at all.

Therapist: Except for making tea sometimes, your husband gives no support.

Caregiver: Yes, yes. My husband is at home, he's retired, and he doesn't support me with caregiving – well, it would be right up my alley if he did though [cynical tone].

Therapist: Well, if I was left to do it all myself, although he's at home and sees what needs to be done – to be honest, I don't think I'd be able to deal with that.

Caregiver: Yes, indeed; it's often difficult for me. It weighs on me, too. He actually goes shopping sometimes, but otherwise he takes the word "retirement" very seriously and doesn't do anything.

Therapist: On top of everything else, this makes your feeling of being left on your own worse and more frustrating.

Caregiver: Yes.

Therapist: You once told me that your sons said to you: "Just put grandpa in a home" ... and that you then felt as though you had to justify yourself. So, you receive hardly any support and encouragement from those around you and then you even have to justify yourself to them about what you do. And now I actually have another hypothesis for you. Maybe it doesn't apply to you at all, but would you like to hear it?

Caregiver: Mm-hmm.

Therapist: Maybe it's a bit like you want to show the others that you can manage to do everything, and this attitude motivates and drives you to continue the care.

Caregiver: Mm-hmm, yes. You are right ... this is often the case. At work it's similar: While others split up work between at least three people, they often leave me to work by myself, because I have proven many times that this works for me ... even when it's so exhausting, I always pull through.

Therapist: Mm-hmm, mm-hmm. Okay ... So that's a heavy burden, if it's always assumed that you will manage and that you must always show others that you can manage.

Caregiver: Yes

Therapist: Let me sum up again: We have just found the path – or part of it – of where your idea comes from that you want to or should take care of your father at home until the end. You said that it's a given in your family that parents and grandparents should be taken care of at home until the end. And now you are taking on this legacy, but with the big difference being that you are in a completely different life situation. You are completely left on your own, your husband doesn't support you, and others are more likely to say, "Put grandpa in a home." There aren't four of you, as was the case with your grandpa. You are completely on your own with everything. Make yourself fully aware of what that means, of all the burden that you are carrying, and also what you are demanding from yourself.

Case Example 11. Responsibility for the person with dementia's well-being

The following excerpt stems from therapy with a 62-year-old caregiving daughter.

Caregiver: It's incredibly hard for me to tell my mother that I'm not there sometimes. I always end up apologizing. At the second attempt, I told her that we're playing tennis for a few days, and it always comes across a bit apologetic. I actually apologized to her for placing her in short-term care.

Therapist: Mm-hmm.

Caregiver: Actually, I don't want to; to apologize for that again. We had already practiced different ways for me to handle the situation, but when I see her sitting there and looking so sad, I feel the need to say something to apologize.

Therapist: On a scale from zero to ten, how strongly do you feel responsible for your mother's happiness? Ten means: "I feel very responsible for my mother's happiness" and zero means: "I don't feel responsible for my mother's happiness or well-being."

Caregiver: Well, I do feel responsible. I once said to you, uh, I remember it exactly: "I am not dependent on my mother's happiness."

Therapist: We even wrote that down, didn't we?

Caregiver: Yes, we even wrote that down.

Therapist: Yes.

Caregiver: But if you ask me like that, I would say that I feel responsible for her well-being. Like between, well ... eight.

Therapist: And has that always been the case? If you think back to the time when you were a young woman and your mother was still living in F.: Did you, would you say that you always felt – well, at that time already – responsible for your mother's well-being and happiness?

Caregiver: Yes.

Therapist: Mm-hmm.

Caregiver: And probably even a ten on the scale. That may have ... it started unconsciously when my father died – well, I was in my late 20s – and she seemed so helpless.

Therapist: Mm-hmm.

Caregiver: And ... it built up because, in hindsight, I sometimes think that she, also took advantage of the fact that I felt so responsible ... yeah, for her well-being, I still feel responsible for that today, I think. I would say eight. Maybe not ten anymore.

Therapist: And when you look at your daughter: How responsible do you think she feels that you're doing well, on a scale from one to ten?

Caregiver: Hmm, what a question, yes [short laughter]. That's difficult for me to answer.

Therapist: Mm-hmm.

Caregiver: I think, I think it would be important to her, but I would say that she does feel responsible, but rather in the lower part of the scale.

Therapist: Mm-hmm, it either makes a difference whether the well-being of your loved one is important to you or whether you feel responsible for it.

Caregiver: Yes.

Therapist: So, you would say that you are important to your daughter, but the responsibility she feels for your well-being would be at the lower end of the scale.

Caregiver: Mm-hmm.

Therapist: And would you say that's healthy like that?

Caregiver: I would find that healthy.

Therapist: Yes.

Caregiver: I have no problem with that, with my daughter.

Therapist: So, you wouldn't demand her to make sure that you're doing well?

Caregiver: No, she once said to me … maybe a year or two ago or longer: "You take a lot of care of grandma, I think that's okay, but you're not responsible for her entertainment. That's her own responsibility. And I wouldn't do that for you guys, either. I would take care of problems that I can solve, but everyone is responsible for their own entertainment" … That was on my mind a lot. I thought then, yes, actually, she's not wrong.

Therapist: Yes.

Caregiver: Otherwise, it's a 100 percent job, which isn't even possible.

Therapist: Okay!

Caregiver: And back then, when the disease had not yet been identified, and she often demanded that I do this or that, it was sometimes too much. You then of course do without – you get used to it and then do without this or that.

Therapist: Mm-hmm.

Caregiver: But, it's probably not right, it's just how I am. It hasn't always been easy in the past and I was really frustrated and angry at times. But now the aspect of the disease is there too, and now I have pity, a strong feeling of compassion for her.

Therapist: Mm-hmm.

Caregiver: And now she's old and sick, and I just want to help, as much … as is within my power.

Therapist: Mm-hmm, and that's what you're doing!

Caregiver: But not, if I …

Therapist: And that's what you're doing!

Caregiver: Yes, no, but it shouldn't go too far; I just can't accept that … I also have a family and to be fair, they need me too.

Therapist: Of you, no?

Caregiver: Of me. And sometimes I feel so hard pressed, because I think that … I won't be able to do this forever.

Therapist: Mm-hmm.

Caregiver: I have a husband who would like to do more things together. This has never been the case before, it was never so obvious. My husband worked a lot, and was away regularly on business trips. … And now, I'll say, my husband demands what he wants. My husband doesn't put it that way, but I notice that he's just … sad when I cancel things. Then I feel like I'm caught in the middle.

Therapist: Would it help you then to weigh up: "What's important to me now at this point? What is more in line with my needs now?"

Caregiver: Yes, the answer is actually clear. Of course, I would like to do something with my husband and with my friends.

Therapist: That's what you want?

Caregiver: That's what I want, and I'm very sure of that.

8.2.2 Imagination Exercises for the Identification and Modification of Dysfunctional Thoughts

In addition to the presented questioning technique, the therapist can also work with specific imagery techniques. This method can be used to guide caregivers to imagine the problem situation vividly, and meanwhile to pay attention to thoughts and feelings. Afterward, instruction is given to review the thoughts or to change the thoughts directly in the imagined situation. With the method of positive imaging, for example, caregivers imagine the situation with already-modified and helpful thoughts and behavior. Case Example 12 illustrates the psycho-imaginative approach, which can immediately provoke significant feelings and encourage the caregivers' reflection process in an effective way ("aha moment"). In the excerpt from a therapy session, the therapist suggests questioning a problematic family agreement by using an imaginative exercise. The family had discussed that no medical treatment should be taken in the event of an emergency or illness of the person with dementia. This agreement was made in order not to disturb the assumed natural dying process and thus to prevent potentially tortuous life-extending medical procedures.

8.2.3 Working Out Effects on Dysfunctional Thoughts on Mood and Behavior

Ellis's (1977) ABC model is suited for explaining and illustrating the effect of dysfunctional thoughts on mood and behavior (see Psychoeducation 3). In this model, activating events, appraisals, and beliefs about the event are linked to emotional and behavioral consequences.

The therapist can use this intervention for main problem areas identified in the initial consultation or for dysfunctional thoughts that are expressed by a caregiver in the sessions. In the first step of this form of cognitive restructuring, caregivers are asked to imagine a problematic situation as vividly as possible. In doing so, occurring thoughts are noted, and their effects on one's own feelings and behavior are analyzed and written down.

Psychoeducation 3. Explanation of the ABC model

> *Therapist:* Surely you're wondering what "ABC" means. I would like to explain this to you now using the situation that we've just written down (discussed): A stands for a particular event or situation, B stands for your perception and beliefs of this event, and C stands for the reaction, for example the thoughts, feelings, and actions that follow the event.

Case Example 12. Burdensome family agreement

The following excerpt stems from therapy with a 58-year-old caregiving daughter.

Therapist: Okay, then I thought in the wrong direction earlier when you said that Christmas will be quite exhausting. I thought about your requirements which you want to meet, to entertain and engage your father at Christmas, but there's something else that resonates, that something life-threatening could happen.

Caregiver: Yes, that too. That always resonates. That's always there, because my father is very weak. He goes to the bathroom and he might collapse. The challenge is to get some distance, to develop calmness, and to say: "Hey, that's not going to happen, even if it does happen, then it happens."

Therapist: The calmness is in your head.

Caregiver: In my head, I know that 100 percent. Where I don't have it, is in my gut.

Therapist: Yes, yes, I can imagine that. What helps you then? If you take your sister as a role model and say: "Okay, I'll try to push this away and I'm going to assume the positive," or would it be better for you to really paint a picture of a scene in your mind, using your thoughts, and to instruct yourself beforehand on how to behave?

Caregiver: How many times do you think I've already done that? [laughs]

Therapist: Yes, and did it help?

Caregiver: No, so at Christmas I really planned to say to myself in the morning or also in the evening: "Hey, if something happens, then it happens, and if he falls down, then he falls down." That I keep telling that to myself, like a mantra.

Therapist: Maybe we could go a little further and you imagine a bad situation and think about what kind of behavior you would want to show in this specific situation. Which bad situation could happen to your father at Christmas?

Caregiver: A bad situation for me would be if he got up in the middle of the night, falls down, passes out – or not – and I don't know whether or not I should call an ambulance.

Therapist: Yes, so you realize that your father has fallen down.

Caregiver: I realize that.

Therapist: Mm-hmm, are you in the same or in a different room?

Caregiver: In another room, but we both have our doors open. Actually, a pin just has to drop, then I'm suddenly awake.

Therapist: You wake up, okay. You then go over, you see your father lying there, and you're looking at whether he's injured himself right? Or do you stand in the door frame and wait?

Caregiver: No, I go in and take a look right away.

Therapist: You go in?

Caregiver: Yes, of course.

Therapist: Mm-hmm. Well, the other alternative would be – according to the agreement that you made with your family – to just simply wait, right?

Caregiver: No. I couldn't stand that. That is not the agreement. The only thing that we agreed on is to wait in terms of calling an ambulance.

Therapist: To wait longer.

Caregiver: Well, not that I wouldn't help my father or that I wouldn't be beside him. That's not the agreement, I wouldn't agree to that. I'm not going to stand in the door frame and let … No, I wouldn't do that!

Therapist: Okay, you go in and take a look. What do you check then? What are you looking at?

Caregiver: Just, whether he's injured himself, if he's still responsive. … Yes. And then … if he has injured himself and isn't responsive … then I get into trouble. Then it will have happened. Then I have to consider: "Do you have to do it now, or can I not do it?"

Therapist: Yes, and what would be helpful for you in the situation? Would an inner distance then be necessary? Would it be better if you left the room shortly to make the decision? Do you call someone? What is your course of action?

Caregiver: I haven't been this far [easy laughing]. That's where I got stuck.

Therapist: Exactly, and then your stomach churns if you don't know: What's actually the plan now? So, suppose your father is lying there and is no longer responsive, and the situation you fear is occurring. What would be the first options for action? What options would you have?

Caregiver: Yes, I mean, I have three options: to call no one, to call my sister, or to call emergency services.

Therapist: Yes, okay.

Caregiver: Those three possibilities I would have. Yes, this is difficult now. Well, my cousin gave me a really good tip and said: "Then just call emergency services. They talk to you first anyway and want to hear what's going on and whether they need to come at all." That might be an alternative that I would have to talk to my family about.

Therapist: So, that you would describe exactly the situation on the telephone ...

Caregiver: Exactly, and that takes 10 or 15 minutes. And that's the problem.

Therapist: Yes, that can be.

Caregiver: Exactly, and that is why it is the case that I already crap my pants just by simply thinking about the situation and my responsibility in that situation. I already paint the whole picture, but then I think: "That's so stupid. Nothing has to happen."

It's good that you're telling me: "Now, go into the situation and think it through to the end." I've never actually thought it through to the end before.

Therapist: It's important to think the situation through to the end, because otherwise anxiety will always resurface. It still doesn't feel great afterward, but you have gone through the situation completely. And you just said that you would have three options. And then you first mentioned the one with the emergency doctor. So, this is the tendency you're gravitating toward?

Caregiver: Hmm, yes, yes. I gravitate toward that, but then I suddenly get the feeling: "Well, you're being a coward, just face it, somehow! You can still do that for your father." And the other thing is: "Well, you've got to do it that way, because you can't really gauge whether this is a short-term thing or if he wants to die now."

Therapist: Yes. Do you actually know your father's position on this?

[...]

Caregiver: Basically, right now I wouldn't necessarily subscribe to the statement that he doesn't want to live anymore.

Therapist: Okay, that of course doesn't make it easier for you.

Caregiver: Exactly, and then I'm not sure: Does he want to go on or not? For *me*, from my way of thinking, I would say: I wouldn't want to go on anymore. Or – I'll elucidate it – *we* will no longer feel like it, if he comes out of the hospital and ends up becoming fully dependent on nursing care. I think, to say it precisely: We won't feel like dealing with it. Then.

Therapist: Mm-hmm. Then.

Caregiver: That might sound hard, but it's ... it hits the nail on the head, I think, quite well. I'm not able to tell anymore what my father is thinking. I can only assume how he might have felt before the onset of his dementia, and I think: "He wouldn't have wanted this."

Therapist: That's right. It's likely that your and your family's suffering is greater than your father's.

Caregiver: Exactly. I think that's exactly what it's all about. I now realize that we are actually the ones saying: "That's only good for him if he then ... no longer goes to the hospital and no longer ..." Because each time he got out of the hospital he was a bit more beside himself than before. Each time a little bit more.

Therapist: Yes, so, by talking about the three possibilities you would have in an emergency situation, we came to the question: Who wants what? Your father would decide differently, probably.

Caregiver: Maybe. I don't know.

Therapist: We don't know.

[...]

Therapist: So, now we've kind of done a walkthrough and addressed different things. What has been important for you today?

Caregiver: I found it very important to think through to the end the situation of my father falling and lying on the floor.

> *Therapist:* That you thought the situation through to the end?
>
> *Caregiver:* Yes. I still have to do a little bit of soul searching and think about it more that we are actually the ones who think: "This isn't working anymore. You let him die now." Actually, I have to say to my family: "Look, I've thought about it, maybe we're actually the ones who want to get rid of him." So, for me this has been very insightful. Maybe that will help me for the decision, *in case* this situation should really occur.
>
> *Therapist:* Mm-hmm, that would be great if that helps you.

The assumption now is that it's not the event itself [use individual example of the caregiver] that produces the reaction [use individual example of the caregiver], but rather your perception and beliefs (B) about the situation [use individual example of the caregiver]. So, it's not the event themselves that trouble you, but rather your appraisal of the event can cause problems and trigger burdensome feelings. Such feelings make us feel uncomfortable and are often at odds with the goals we're aiming for. Furthermore, these feelings often make the situation worse.

With the aid of the ABC model, it is explained to the caregivers that the way they appraise an event has an impact on their physical and mental state and on their experience of burden (see Case Example 13). The therapist asks the caregiver to describe a stressful situation, using Worksheet 8-1: ABC Model, and to write it down if necessary. These questions can be helpful for this process:
- In which situation did the thought arise (when, where, who, what)?
- Remember exactly what went through your mind in this situation.
- Which expectations and beliefs did you have?
- How did you feel during and after?
- Which positive or negative consequences did the thought have?
- What did you do or avoid?
- Can you remember your bodily reactions?

As a therapeutic task between sessions, caregivers are asked to observe themselves in stressful situations, noting occurring thoughts and emotional consequences in a thought diary and listening to their mind as if they had a "third ear." In this way, caregivers are increasingly sensitized to recognize their own dysfunctional thoughts and motivated to question them.

Subsequently, with the help of the technique of Socratic dialogue, dysfunctional thoughts are questioned and alternative thoughts are developed. Finally, caregivers are then asked to write down the alternative, helpful thoughts on a notecard and to place the notecard in a visible place as a frequent reminder.

In the next session experiences with the ABC model are discussed and possible problems or questions that may arise are clarified.

Please note

Especially in the case of dementia caregiving, it is sometimes not enough to develop alternative thoughts or appraisals with caregivers. In addition, therapists need to help with the search for specific solutions. Interventions such as problem analysis and problem solving, as described in Chapter 9, can be helpful and necessary.

The cognitive restructuring technique is one of the central interventions of therapeutic work with caregivers and is used accordingly for almost all topics presented in this manual. In summary, through cognitive restructuring caregivers learn to recognize debilitating and discouraging thoughts and to develop alternative, potentially stress-reducing and encouraging thoughts. Emphasis should also be placed on tasks between sessions in which the caregivers are asked to observe themselves in stressful situations and write down occurring thoughts and emotional consequences in a thought diary. In this way, they will be increasingly sensitized to recognize their own dysfunctional thoughts and motivated to question them and replace them with more helpful ones. Applying and writing down these self-developed, helpful thoughts in everyday situations enables caregivers to experience the positive changes that more helpful thoughts can have on their own perception and behavior.

Case Example 13. Always having to be there for the ill person

The following excerpt stems from therapy with a 76-year-old caregiving wife.

Caregiver: My son knows caregivers who are off at least once a month. And he says to me: "With all due respect, you should be able to make that happen too." But I wasn't thrilled at all.

Therapist: Yes, I believe that. Take the ABC model again; I think the situation fits quite well. The situation is that you were away for 2 hours, came back and saw that your husband was sitting there and happy that you were back. What was going through your mind?

Caregiver: There wasn't much going through my mind, but through my heart – how nice that he's so happy.

Therapist: You just insinuated something else, which is that it's not easy for you to leave, because you think: "Maybe he's not doing well if I'm not there."

Caregiver: Although, when I ask him if I can leave longer, he says, "Yes": He wants me to do something nice. But he's not doing very well.

Therapist: How do you notice that?

Caregiver: From the joy. But maybe that's not the case. He also takes a nap and sleeps, is not restless, he talks to the bird.

Therapist: And how do you think he is feeling?

Caregiver: He's not doing badly, but he misses me. But that's something else, that he misses me and that he's doing badly. I don't really think he's doing badly.

Therapist: How are you doing now, when you say it like that?

Caregiver: I'm doing better.

Therapist: Then you have successfully done the ABC model! That he misses you is something different than him not doing well; as a result, you feel better. So, in situations in which you are not doing so well, you might think: Is this really the case, or are there maybe other explanations?

Caregiver: Yes, I could do that.

Therapist: How could one find out now if it would be okay for your husband to have someone come and help with care so that you could do more for yourself?

Caregiver: Mm-hmm, good question.

Therapist: So far, only you have provided care?

Caregiver: When he had his operation, nurses also came into the house. He accepted them well. Perhaps one should just try it, quite simply. I get the impression that I'm worrying too much.

Therapist: Have you ever experienced that it is very helpful to try things out?

Caregiver: Yes, quite often actually.

Therapist: Okay, that's great! I would like to give you a small homework assignment. I would like to ask you to choose a specific day on which you can do something for yourself and to prepare everything you need in order to do so.

9 "You Are Still at Home Here!" – Dealing With Challenging Behavior

Family caregivers often experience ambivalent feelings regarding the behavior of the person with dementia. On the one hand, there exists knowledge that the disease involves changes in personality and behavior; on the other hand, however, there are also phases of incomprehension or helplessness toward problem behaviors. It is demanding for the caregiver to comprehend the person with dementia's behavior as part of the disease, because the symptoms are sometimes fluctuating, unpredictable, or simply not understandable.

One typical symptom of dementia is memory impairment, namely forgetfulness, and, associated with this, constantly repeating oneself or asking questions. Other behaviors caused by the disease, such as aggressive behavior or making accusations, are more difficult to attribute to dementia clearly and to distinguish from intentional behavior. For the caregiver, this often leads to negative interpretations of the person rather than attributions to the illness and/or the corresponding situation. Therefore, persons with dementia are sometimes described as uncomprehending, egocentric, inattentive, unreasonable, complaining, accusatory, hurtful, and not adhering to the rules. Accordingly, family members react with anger, irritability, fear, fury, powerlessness, emotional detachment, and helplessness. Case Example 14, of a caregiving granddaughter, illustrates the problem in which caregivers often find themselves.

When asked about the most burdensome changes, family members report very heterogeneous behaviors. Table 4 lists examples of behaviors that family caregivers typically experience as being very disruptive.

9.1 Goals of the Module

When dealing with difficult behaviors, it is helpful to assume that the person with dementia's behavioral changes are due to the illness. The point is to align knowledge about the illness with corresponding appraisals and actions. This is, in many cases, very difficult for family members. A therapeutic goal is to understand, assume, and accept challenging behaviors (see also the concept of validation by Feil & de Klerk-Rubin, 2015). It is not uncommon for difficult behaviors to result in unfavora-

---

Case Example 14. Between knowledge and incomprehension

The following excerpt stems from therapy with a 31-year-old caregiving granddaughter.

Caregiver: I've read a lot and, in my head, I know that it's the dementia and what one has to do, 100 percent or 80 percent.

Therapist: Only "your gut" sometimes says something else?

Caregiver: Yes, pretty much. Sometimes I'm not quite sure. Because on some days she manages well, on other days nothing works. Then I think that she should just put forth a little more effort. I then have little understanding for her behavior. I often get angry in such situations.

Therapist: What do you get angry about?

Caregiver: Because I just don't want to admit to myself that she can't do many things anymore. One always thinks: "She just doesn't want to." But that's nonsense! It's just nonsense.

Table 4. Examples of challenging behaviors

Physically aggressive behavior	Yes, and then he becomes really mean, because he doesn't recognize anything at all and then he tries to hit me.
Verbally aggressive behavior	I can't really deal with her yelling at me. I then go home and think about it for days. She then says, for example, "You bitch, you bastard, you dirty rat!" She lays it on the line. The expressions I hear hurt me severely.
Unrest and vocal disturbances (e.g., loud shouting)	My husband is often very restless in the morning. Then he shouts loudly and walks around in the other rooms.
Constantly asking questions, repeating oneself	My mother asks all day: "When can I go home?" "When will I be picked up?" always the same. I can explain to her 10 times that she is at home here. A minute later she asks me again.
Wandering, e.g., with the goal of going home	He always wants to go out in the evening. When we sit there and watch TV, he says, "Now we're going home." Then he gets up and wants to go. When I've then said three or four times: "You are at home here. Sit down," he says again, "Now we're going home." And then he gets going again.
Depressive mood, passive behavior, apathy, withdrawal behavior	What bothers me the most is that he just sits there and does nothing and is so apathetic. When he does that, I want to run away. He has become quiet, he speaks very little. He is no longer interested in anything. When he does say something, it's mostly negative.
Defensive/resistance behavior	Sometimes I have the feeling that he does it on purpose. He also has such a childish mind, a "spirit of contradiction" that one experiences with small children. He always takes it up a notch, no matter what I do.
Accusations	What bothers me a lot is the bad-mouthing and accusations. For example, her flowers have wilted. She wouldn't say though that her flowers have wilted, but that one of us has ripped them out.
Clingy behavior or shadowing	It bothers me that he's constantly behind me. For example, if I got up now to go to the bathroom, he would stand in front of the bathroom door and wait until I got out of the bathroom. I can't walk anywhere, down any hallway, do anything alone anymore.
Special habits, e.g., throwing things away or hoarding	It bothers me that he now has the habit of throwing everything away. He even threw away his dentures, and we didn't even notice.
Socially inappropriate behavior, not following rules	It bothers me when he uses my towel! I say to him: "Hey, that's my towel!" Then he says, "I can use it, I'm your husband!" He never did that in the past. And when I then say, "I don't like that" he then says again: "I'm your husband and I can do that! We are one!" After that, I say "No. This has nothing to do with that. I don't want this!" And then he gets stubborn and does it anyway.
Incontinence	I understand if he forgets, that's his illness, but that's no reason to be so dirty. I scold him, when he's made a mess in his pants. I say: "Look at this! What have you done again?" And then he says: "I can't see anything" or, "It wasn't me!" Then I say, "I know that it was you!"

ble patterns of interaction, which can cause feelings of shame and anger among family members. The better the knowledge and understanding of dementia-related behaviors, the easier it is to develop appropriate interaction strategies and reduce feelings of shame and anger. To achieve this, occurring behaviors are analyzed, and helpful strategies for dealing with difficult behaviors are imparted. In addition, to facilitate understanding, necessary information on the disease and its course is explained.

In this chapter, a list of "universal" problem-solving strategies is explicitly omitted, since the individual family caregiver's situations differ too greatly to be able to present an adequate solution for each situation. Box 11 contains an overview of the interventions covered in this chapter.

Box 11. Overview of the interventions

- Psychoeducation and guided discovery
- Exploring challenging behaviors and encouraging self-disclosure
- Problem analysis of challenging behaviors using microanalyses
- Changing dysfunctional and encouraging alternative appraisals
- Problem-solving techniques

9.2 Therapeutic Approach

9.2.1 Psychoeducation and Guided Discovery

Information on problem behaviors of persons with dementia is particularly important because clinical experience shows that many family members attribute these behaviors not to dementia, but to the personality of the person affected or various other causes, such as age. Family members should thus be informed about challenging behaviors that are caused in relation to the disease (see also Chapter 3). Box 12 shows topics for which information sheets are available (Worksheet 9-1 to Worksheet 9-17 in the Appendix). Further information is offered in the guide "Caring for a Person With Dementia: A Practical Guide" (Alzheimer's Society UK, 2022). In addition to the topics listed here, it also contains information on other difficult behaviors.

Box 12. Topics on the worksheets (see Appendix)

1. General Tips for Dealing With Difficult Behaviors (Worksheet 9-1)
2. Wandering Around Aimlessly (Worksheet 9-2)
3. Restlessness, Sleep–Wake–Rhythm Disorders (Worksheet 9-3)
4. Constant Questions, Repeating Oneself (Worksheet 9-4)
5. Anxiety (Worksheet 9-5)
6. Accusations, Distrust (Worksheet 9-6)
7. Unfavorable Habits I: Throwing Important Things Away (Worksheet 9-7)
8. Unfavorable Habits II: Searching, Rummaging, Collecting, Hoarding (Worksheet 9-8)
9. Incontinence (Worksheet 9-9)
10. Personal Hygiene (Worksheet 9-10)
11. Feelings of Disgust (Worksheet 9-11)
12. Eating and Drinking (Worksheet 9-12)
13. Problems With Visits to the Doctor (Worksheet 9-13)
14. Driving (Worksheet 9-14)
15. Safety Precautions (Worksheet 9-15)
16. Behavior Analysis (Worksheet 9-16)
17. Behavior Experiment Protocol (Worksheet 9-17)

The worksheets contain general information on how to deal with various difficult behaviors and serve as a basis for discussion. They should be adapted individually to the current life situation of the family. As the exemplary overview of the structure of an information sheet shows, the problem situation and possible causes are listed on one side, and what the relatives can do to cope with the situation on the other side.

In particular, it should be discussed with the caregivers to what extent they themselves contribute to the development and preservation of the person with dementia's behaviors. Problem behaviors occur, for example, through the person with dementia's confrontation with difficult-to-manage situations or through inadvertent criticism, personal offence, uncertainty, and excessive demands from the family members and/or the environment (Haupt, 1999; Kurz, 1998). Since the affected persons frequently do not understand the family caregivers sufficiently and, in many cases, can no longer clearly communicate their own thoughts, needs, wishes, and feelings, they react with anxiety or with aggression as a form of self-protection (Feil, 2012; Höwler, 2008; Wilz et al., 2001). Moreover, the perception of the loss of competence, such as not being able to dress oneself alone, can trigger feelings of shame and frustration, which can lead to unpredictable behavioral reactions. It is very helpful to impart to the caregivers that a stance that encourages the person with dementia's autonomy as much as possible usually improves their own quality of life and that of the person with dementia. Example 11 shows a simple, creative solution that makes it easier for the person with dementia to accept the aid of a wheelchair.

Example 11. Creative problem solving: Strengthening the self-esteem of the person with dementia

> *Caregiver:* He has had a wheelchair since Monday. But it's his taxi and not a wheelchair. I hadn't thought of that. That is what the nurse said. She said to me: "M., don't call it a wheelchair, then he won't want to sit in it! Say 'taxi' instead, and then it's kind of …"
>
> *Therapist:* Great!
>
> *Caregiver:* Right?! She's pretty clever.
>
> *Therapist:* I like it, yes.

Family caregivers who have knowledge of the causes of the person with dementia's behavior benefit with respect to these important aspects: They have more understanding for the patient, experience relief, and can develop appropriate behavior in dealing with the patient. Psychoeducation 4 shows the importance of encouraging activity and autonomy in the person with dementia.

Psychoeducation 4. Encouraging activity and autonomy of the patient

> *Therapist:* Yes, that's too bad when the fruit dries out, or the cheese gets dry. I can understand that. But I think that it has to do with the fact that she is happy that, as you say, this is one of the things that she can still manage on her own, where she notices, it still works: "I'm preparing something, I'm making myself useful." She's prepared a meal and is looking forward to you coming home. Although you've tried to talk to her about it and have said, "We can do this together," it seems like this is very important to her, and she forgets what you've said. And perhaps it's really about you cherishing the moment and accepting it and overlooking the dried cheese.
>
> *Caregiver:* Yes, well, that's not what really bothers me, but you realize that you think everything's working out, then you see that that's not really the case.
>
> *Therapist:* Yes, those are the small signs here and there. But it's important that you actually praise her and encourage her existing skills that she can still do. If you get the impression that an ability has been lost, don't try to rebuild it or train it, because in most cases, that won't work. If the ability is gone, it tends to make the person with dementia feel even more incompetent. Instead, encourage what still works, for example setting the table. Even if it doesn't always work out how you want it to. I wouldn't spend a lot of energy discussing that with her over and over again, but say: "Nice, I'm glad you've done that," even if you're secretly a little upset.

Case Example 15 will clarify how the therapist helps the caregiver better understand the illness by using guided discovery. Consequently, the caregiver realizes that she has asked too much of her husband suffering from dementia in some situations. The newly acquired knowledge about the illness helps the caregiver to be able to deal with the person with dementia more calmly and no longer behave in a demanding, offensive, and insulting manner. The person with dementia is then less likely to experience failure, which in turn fosters their self-esteem and autonomy.

9.2.2 Exploring Challenging Behaviors and Encouraging Self-Disclosure

It is helpful to talk and ask questions about the caregiving situation and symptoms to gather challenging behaviors. Here it is important to create a foundation of trust that enables caregivers to speak openly about the person with dementia's behavior and the caregiving situation. Initially, it is very difficult for some caregivers to talk about behaviors of the person with dementia that are assessed as shameful and/or about their own reactions in the caregiving context. Questions 9 can be helpful for this exploration.

Questions 9. Exploring challenging behaviors

> - How has your family member changed since the illness?
> - Can you describe your family member's personality and has it changed due to the illness?
> - Which behavioral changes or problems bother you the most?
> - Can you describe in more detail a situation in which the behavior recently occurred?
> - When, where, and how often does this behavior occur?

Case Example 15. Guided discovery to encourage understanding the person with dementia

The following excerpt stems from therapy with a 75-year-old caregiving wife.

Therapist: What do you think helped you react more calmly in the situation?

Caregiver: Yes, certainly our talks. They certainly contributed to the fact that I react a little more mellow – even before the situation.

Therapist: And do you have an idea of *what* made you more detached?

Caregiver: I think the reason is that I can better classify the disease and his condition. You advised me to imagine a pearl necklace when he doesn't get everything sorted in the bathroom in the morning, and, and … everything that we have discussed.

Therapist: Okay, that means you see the disease from a different perspective and imagine certain images like the pearl necklace, which contains pearls of different sizes that create a certain pattern. And now, similar to how your husband's memory is no longer sorted, the pearls are no longer strung in a particular order – this image helped you to understand your husband's behavior.

Caregiver: Now I write down more things for him. Not like in the past, when I asked him for example to write down five countries as a task. I don't do that anymore. I also read that this is not necessarily a good thing because it shows him quite plainly what his limitations are when he is no longer able to manage a certain situation. No, I mean, I write down for him how he has to put on his pants. At night, he doesn't go out of the room at all. And if he slightly wets himself, then he changes his pants. Then, quite often he asks: "In the back is the fly, in the front the label, right?" And then we would have discussion after discussion, and now I've written it down for him and since then it works.

Therapist: And how did you write it down for him?

Caregiver: Now he has a notebook lying in the bedroom and in it I wrote: "Label always in the back" and marked it with a red pen.

Therapist: That's great that it works, isn't it? I would still like to talk about one aspect, specifically, why's it so bad for you when he puts his pants on backward?

Caregiver: Uh, well, men's pants are made so that there is a lot more space in the front than in the back. That's … Maybe it's not so comfortable or it will pinch or what do I know, and then he won't tell me – but it's possible.

Therapist: Has he ever said anything like that?

Caregiver: No, not really. Well, nobody sees it except me in the morning. But, I mean, now I have clarified it, now I don't have to think anymore about whether he puts his pants on backward or not.

Therapist: It's possible now though that at some point he won't be able to read things or understand their meaning anymore. That's something that can come with the progression of the disease.

Caregiver: Well, then I would have to [exhaling deeply] stop criticizing that with the pants. Then that's just the way it is. But let me say: just so long as it works.

Therapist: If you had the idea and it works, then that's great. My question was aimed at, what would happen if it doesn't work anymore: What's so bad about his pants being worn backward?

Caregiver: In principle, nothing, if he doesn't say: "It's pinching" or "They don't fit" or something like that. Yes, I didn't plan on the possibility of that happening at some point. I always go from … the actual state, I'd say. But if you say that this can happen to us, that later he may not be able to read or swallow …

Therapist: I don't want to scare you.

Caregiver: Actually, I know this, I've read it. But I have never taken it into account for myself.

Therapist: Sometimes changes or impairments can come very suddenly. Nothing can change for a long time, but then something changes strongly. This is very irregular, one cannot predict the course of this illness. And that's why I asked you, because it *can* happen. It doesn't have to though. And it's great that you've thought about the situation and tried something new. It worked and that's great. To the question, what would be so bad if he puts his pants on backward, you said: "Well, that wouldn't be so bad." My only thought now is whether it wouldn't relieve you a little bit to know that it wouldn't be so bad for you.

Caregiver: I don't know now either, but in the nursing home it seems that the nurses' tactic is that they overlook certain things. And when I spoke to the manager, he said that they don't take things like that so seriously anyway. When the dementia patients feel like they have to put on two shirts, then they just let them put on two shirts. And I didn't really like that.

Therapist: What bothers you about that?

Caregiver: Yes, that they don't care how they walk around. And I mean, when … It's probably different when you're with your family, isn't it?

Therapist: I'm glad that you mentioned this. You also read that it is not so good to always draw someone's attention to their mistakes. You had just put it that way, did I understand you correctly?

Caregiver: Yes, of course. He doesn't even always realize his shortcomings.

Therapist: Exactly. And it's the same with the other things. If you tell your husband: "Jeez, you have your pants on backward again" then he will be confronted with his flaw at this moment. Or if someone has put on two shirts and then you say: "Jeez, you put on two shirts – you did it wrong again! You should put on only one!" then at that moment it's the same. One will be confronted with their flaw. This means that, as a caregiver if you, like the manager of the nursing home – I'll say – ignore it, or just leave it as the patient does it, does that then automatically mean that you're not providing enough care?

Caregiver: No, not in that case. But I got the impression.

Therapist: Ah, okay.

Caregiver: When I handle it like this, my husband lives more calmly, and so do I. Is that the same thing then? Yes, I didn't think that far again. I only saw: "How are they letting people walk around?" That's just not how I am.

Therapist: And you're doing a lot and you take care of him well. You keep an eye on your husband so well that it's not a sign of you providing bad care if he has his underpants on backward.

Caregiver: Yes, and nobody would notice at that moment, because he doesn't run around in his underpants when there is a visitor.

Therapist: Sometimes you can ask yourself the question: "What is more important to me at this moment? Is it more important that he uses the right towel, for example, or is it more important that I leave him his independence as much as possible? Leave him to his own rules and/or his own self-worth, without making it clear to him again, "Jeez, you made a mistake again!" This has both advantages and disadvantages. "If I confront him with his mistakes, that will …" Well, what is the disadvantage of that? Can you imagine what that would be?

Caregiver: Yes, then his self-esteem is hurt.

Therapist: And, on the other hand, to endure for yourself that he may have dabbed his face with the wrong towel has the disadvantage for you, so to speak, or for your husband that it may not be so hygienic. But the advantage is: His feeling of self-worth isn't chipped away at. This means that we actually always have advantages and disadvantages for both decision possibilities.

Caregiver: Yes, that's true, mm-hmm.

Therapist: Just like … just like the head nurse acted.

Caregiver: I, I ... As I said, I couldn't really understand it then. I thought: "The head nurse, it doesn't matter to him what they do," but now it's been put into perspective when I think about it using your observations. Yes [deep exhale], that's why we're doing this, so that I can look a little behind it, right?

Therapist: What exactly are you remembering for yourself now?

Caregiver: When I signed up for therapy, I always tried to instruct him and convert him, and he was broken and I was done.

Therapist: You were pretty burdened there, right?

Caregiver: Yes! And then I had read about the study and thought: "You're just going to try this now," and I find that one is able to grow better, in dealing with it. Surely there are sometimes situations where I then react incorrectly again. I don't always react correctly. That also happens.

Therapist: Of course that happens. And that's allowed to happen, Mrs. M., because you're not a machine, right? You're a human.

Caregiver: Yeah [exhales], that's clear, but generally, I'll say, I can handle it differently now.

Furthermore, information on the frequency, duration, and intensity should be collected. It should be taken into consideration that the behaviors are subject to fluctuations and change throughout the course of the disease. It should also be noted that problem behaviors vary in different forms of dementia (see Halek & Bartholomeyczik, 2006). If caregivers mention several behaviors that are experienced as disturbing, it is advisable to explore these in succession.

In addition to burdensome behavior, the context in which the behavior occurs should be covered in detail. This is because the context affects the person with dementia's behavior and interactions. Therefore, it is important to examine the context closely in order to clarify the source and causes of the challenging behaviors. The use of behavioral analyses is suitable for considering the context conditions and for analyzing the triggering and maintaining factors. How to apply behavioral analyses will be described in Section 9.2.3.

9.2.3 Behavioral Analysis

Within the context of several specific behavioral analyses on the microlevel, the following should be addressed: how the caregiver reacts to challenging behavior in a specific situation, how they appraise and processes this, and, in turn, which consequences their behavior has for the person with dementia. Questions 10 lists examples of helpful questions for analyzing a specific problem situation.

Questions 10. Analyzing context conditions for a specific problem behavior

- Does this behavior also occur in other contexts, for example in the day-care facility? What is different there? What is different at home?
- Does your relative show this behavior in front of other people as well?
- How is their behavior when dealing with other people?
- Are there times when this behavior doesn't occur?
- Did your family member show this behavior before they became ill?
- Who is involved?
- What happens before the disturbing behavior?

Case Example 16 illustrates how the problem analysis procedure can be explained to the caregiver.

The problem analyses compiled with the caregivers can be transferred to Worksheet 9-16: Behavior Analysis, for better presentation and clarity.

For complex, extremely burdensome problem situations, analyzing the challenging behavior requires a detailed dialogue with the caregivers. In several steps, triggering factors, context conditions, reactions of the caregivers, and behavioral consequences are worked out. The session sequence in Case Example 17 shows the analysis of anxiety and delusional symptoms, which are experienced as extremely burdensome and uncontrollable by the family caregiver. Because several challenging behaviors occur in this case example, a longer session segment was chosen to be presented.

Case Example 16. Psychoeducation and problem analysis

The following excerpt stems from therapy with a 61-year-old caregiving husband.

Therapist: What I would like for you to do, Mr. M., is to really consciously observe yourself, to reflect for yourself: Which situations lead to more fury and impatience? In which situations is it harder for you to calm down mentally, and in which situations do you find it easier? Please take out the Behavior Analysis worksheet.

Caregiver: Behavior Analysis.

Therapist: Exactly, and now it's similar to how it was earlier in our talk when I asked you: What is the situation, and how do you react, what's going through your mind? For example, "I've had enough, I have to put her in a home now." One feeling in such a situation is probably anger, and your body also reacts somehow. You might notice your agitation, tension, or your heart beating. And you behave in a certain way, maybe by leaving the situation or scolding your wife and saying: "Now don't make such a fuss like that!" Of course, I don't know exactly what you say in the situation. And all of this of course has consequences. And there are short-term and long-term ones. And we had already worked out that as a consequence you sometimes have feelings of guilt, that you thought something like that, and said to yourself: "Jeez, how could you think such a thing?" And that also has consequences, in terms of how you then behave. And this scheme here on the worksheet is a type of support, so to speak, that you can use to analyze different situations for yourself. And it gives us, I think, a clue as to where you can change something for yourself. So, until our next session, it would be great if you could observe yourself in situations using this scheme, and to take notes and to ponder: "What was going through my head in this situation, that I reacted so angrily, and what was different in the other situation, so that I could calm down a little bit or react to her differently?"

Case Example 17. Behavioral analysis for delusional symptoms and anxiety

The following excerpt stems from therapy with a 61-year-old caregiving husband.

Caregiver: It's very, very difficult. Especially the screaming at night. It's terrible. During the night from Wednesday to Thursday, she screamed "Help!" *For hours.*

Therapist: Yes, could you describe the situation again in more detail? You had told me in our previous sessions that the screaming can last for 1 to 2 hours?

Caregiver: Yes, she gets worked up about something for which she needs help, for example that she's freezing to death or drowning, what do I know ... and then she screams. And it's no use for me to say: "You're still lying in your bed and it's nice and warm. You don't have to freeze to death," but it's no use at all. And now a lion has attacked her or a snake has bitten her. ... And then she gets so worked up and starts screaming.

Therapist: And then she screams for help?

Caregiver: "Help" or "Mom" or also other names that I don't even know anymore. She screams so loudly for them to help her.

Therapist: And how do you react to it? You have just described that you try to calm her down by saying for example that she is in bed and everything is fine.

Caregiver: I then turn on the light. I say: "Look, you're lying in your bed and it's nice and warm, you're not cold at all." And then she starts with me too. That I have to get out too, I'm freezing too. But she's very warm, she's not cold. I even touched her to see if she really was cold. I have no idea what's going on in her head.

Therapist: Yes, that is difficult to figure out, how she's experiencing it and why she has these fears.

Caregiver: And also constantly that she's fallen into the water and is soaking wet – that's also one of the things she gets worked up about. I have to undress her, she's soaking wet. I say to her: "Come on, feel yourself, you're not wet at all." Maybe I'm not reacting properly, I don't know.

Therapist: Yes, so you're trying to help her again and again by telling her it's not what she's experiencing at the moment, but that you tell her that she's taken care of, that she's doing well, isn't drowning and isn't freezing.

Caregiver: Yes, that's what I try.

Therapist: But she can't understand that at that moment.

Caregiver: No, she doesn't accept it. After I tell her that, she screams again. And the loudness: Her voice was very hoarse, she screamed like that all day.

Therapist: How else are you behaving? You said that you first check if she really is wet or cold?

Caregiver: Yes, that's what I tried. I said: "Look, you're completely warm from head to toe; you can't be freezing to death," but it's really no use.

Therapist: And when did the point come where she stopped? Can you understand when and why she stops?

Caregiver: Well, this week, she almost didn't stop at all. I told her in the morning: "I have to work all day, and you kept screaming even though you had promised that you would let me sleep." I tried it that way, because she is always concerned with my well-being. I say: "You have to let me sleep. Otherwise, I won't be able to do this anymore." But that probably doesn't get through to her anymore. When she has yelled herself tired, I think, that's mostly after 1 or 2 hours.

Therapist: So, another strategy of yours was that you play on her always being concerned for your well-being. But that doesn't get through to her at that moment?

Caregiver: No. I said, "Look, you promised me that you would be quiet now so that I can sleep. You promised me that. You always said: 'One has to keep one's promises.'" But 2 minutes later she starts screaming again. And then I thought that the doctor could help me somehow. But he told me he can't help me either.

Therapist: What happens to you then, how are you when your wife starts screaming?

Caregiver: I feel aggressive. You can't take it anymore.

Therapist: That's completely understandable.

Caregiver: So yesterday, I said: "Well, you want to scream and you don't want to stop, then I'll take you to the basement now. And I'll close all the doors there and you can scream in the basement." And then she became really aggressive. When I said "We're going to the basement now and you can scream there as loudly as you want, because nobody will be able to hear you anymore," then I was pooped and she got aggressive. She comes at me and tries to hit me. And that's not a solution. When she's screamed for so long, I'm *so* at the end of my ropes that I could just cry. But that's no use for me either.

Possible solutions for Case Example 16 are presented in Section 9.2.6: Problem-Solving Strategies for Behavior Modification.

9.2.4 Goals for Dealing Better With Challenging Behaviors

After exploring difficult behaviors and analyzing their triggers and maintaining/reinforcing conditions, goals for better dealing with the person with dementia in the future can be discussed.

From a family caregiver's perspective, there are occasionally unrealistic goals. Therefore, the goals formulated together with the caregivers should be reflected upon and checked whether they are realistic and feasible. Example 12 gives an example of unrealistic expectations.

Example 12. Unrealistic expectations of the ill person

Caregiver: It would be much more peaceful, and I would be less emotionally upset or less annoyed, or less disappointed if she occasionally said: "Come on, I realize it. Don't take it the wrong way, I've forgotten, I'm asking you for the seventh time," or something like that.

In such cases, it should be made clear to the caregiver that the person with dementia is usually no longer able to reason coherently. At the same time, more realistic goals should be discussed and reflected upon.

Family caregivers already utilize various cognitive and behavioral strategies to deal with difficult behaviors. In the therapeutic sessions, it should be decided which strategies used by the caregivers for the specific situation appear to be appropriate and advisable and can be evaluated as constructive.

9.2.5 Modification of Appraisals

Another central component is working with cognitive techniques. In doing so, interpretations and causal attributions for the person with dementia's behavior should be questioned. The validity of these assumptions can be checked using Socratic dialogue (see also Chapter 8). Questions 11 lists helpful questions.

Questions 11. Helpful questions for questioning appraisals of challenging behavior

- Which aspects of their behavior are due to dementia?
- What explanations are there for their behavior?
- Do they always behave this way/are there exceptions? When/in which situations do they behave differently?
- Would they behave this way if they were healthy?
- Did they behave this way in the past?

The caregiver's interpretation of the behaviors plays an important role with respect to the experience of burden and can be very different for each individual. For example, some caregivers may hardly evaluate certain behaviors of the person with dementia negatively, while others experience the same behaviors as being very disturbing. Many family caregivers experience great relief by being able to talk about the problematic behaviors. An open and nonjudgmental approach by the therapist is helpful for exploration. This makes it easier for the caregivers to speak about the behaviors openly, as Case Example 18 illustrates.

> **Case Example 18. Accusations "You have other men in bed"**
>
> The following excerpt stems from therapy with a 70-year-old female life partner.
>
> *Caregiver:* Yesterday, he accused me again of having other men in bed under my covers. He says: "Well, how many guys did you invite again?" or "How many are there under your covers, show me!" It gets me down, I can't take it anymore. I don't know where he gets this idea, I simply don't understand it.
>
> *Therapist:* It's really not an easy situation. What goes through your mind the moment he accuses you?
>
> *Caregiver:* Well, I think: "This can't be true, this is outrageous that he's accusing me of such a thing, I never did wrong." It's simply not true.
>
> *Therapist:* Mm-hmm, exactly, and what does that do to you? How does that make you feel?
>
> *Caregiver:* It makes me mad as hell.
>
> *Therapist:* It makes you furious?
>
> *Caregiver:* Yes, it makes me angry. Very much so, and you know, it also makes me extremely sad that he doesn't trust me at all. That he really thinks I have men in bed. He has no reason to think that.
>
> *Therapist:* Yes, you say that it makes you angry and makes you sad. And physically? Do you notice a change there too?
>
> *Caregiver:* Yes, I'm very tense, everything feels cramped somehow.
>
> *Therapist:* Yes, I understand. You are tense, and everything feels cramped. What do you do then? How do you deal with it?
>
> *Caregiver:* Well, to be honest, I yell at him. I say: "Stop with this crap, stop accusing me of such a thing. There's no one here."
>
> *Therapist:* Okay, because it makes you so angry, you yell at him.

Caregiver: Yes, I know that it's not right, but I just can't do anything else at this moment.

Therapist: Yes, I think it's quite an automatic reaction that's happening to you. What are the consequences usually when you yell at him?

Caregiver: He doesn't stop. He continues accusing me, which can last all day, and do you know what the worst part is? He tries to get close to me physically. As if he wants to prove to me that he's the man of the house. And it makes me so uncomfortable, I then turn him away, but then I get the feeling that then he really does think that I have something going on with other men.

Therapist: I find it very understandable that this is very uncomfortable for you. Did I understand you correctly that he doesn't stop if you yell at him and make it clear to him that you don't have any men with you? On the contrary: He then tries to get physically close to you?

Caregiver: Yes. It's no use at all.

Therapist: Yes, to begin with, it doesn't help?

Caregiver: Not really. On the contrary, it just seems to make it worse.

Therapist: That is an important finding. In the next step, we can think about how you might be able to find other ways to deal with the accusations.

Caregiver: Yes, that would be good.

Possible solutions for Case Example 17 are presented in Section 9.2.6: Problem-Solving Strategies for Behavior Modification.

As Case Example 18 shows, dysfunctional appraisals and the resulting feelings lead to further negative consequences for caregivers and the persons with dementia alike. For example, feelings of anger and shame can reinforce avoidance of situations and caregivers' withdrawal behavior. Therefore, the goal is that family caregivers learn to describe their thoughts and feelings and to better understand the effects on the interaction with the person with dementia.

Case Example 19 illustrates how to work on changing caregivers' burdensome thoughts.

Burdensome feelings of shame also often arise if the person with dementia violates social rules and norms (e.g., when going out to eat or in contact with friends), if the caregivers feel embarrassed, and also if they fear losing their social recognition. It is typical for caregivers to feel ashamed not for their own behavior, but for the behavior of the person with dementia. In turn, these feelings of shame lead to avoidance of social situations, for example, dining out together. Moreover, feelings of shame can arise as a consequence of one's own reactions to the person with dementia's behavior.

Through cognitive techniques, family caregivers can be shown alternative interpretations and appraisals that do not trigger feelings of shame and anger and that reduce avoidance (see Example 13).

Example 13. Feelings of shame

> *Caregiver:* My father throws the rest of his food off the balcony, as if no one would live below him. However, his pharmacist lives there. You wouldn't believe how embarrassing this is for me. But the lady is very understanding.

Behavioral experiments

Behavioral experiments (in the context of treatment of social anxiety disorder, according to Stangier et al., 2003, see Psychoeducation 5) can be planned with the caregivers to modify thoughts and to reduce avoidance behavior and can be carried out as transfer exercises. Afterward, the new experiences can be assessed with the caregivers.

First, the caregivers should collect situations in which the shameful behavior is likely to occur. The caregivers are instructed on exactly how they should behave in those situations (e.g., consciously pay attention to how others react). Protocol sheets can be used to prepare and follow up the exercises (see Worksheet 9-17: Behavior Experiment Protocol).

> **Case Example 19. Changing burdensome appraisals**
>
> The following excerpt stems from therapy with a 45-year-old caregiving daughter.
>
> *Therapist:* You reported that it's very difficult for you that your father keeps packing his suitcase, because he thinks that he's going on a journey.
>
> *Caregiver:* Exactly, it's just totally exhausting for me, because I keep having to empty out everything. And he does it over and over again and I've explained to him so many times that he's not traveling anywhere. I say: "Dad, stop it now, you're not going anywhere, you haven't traveled anywhere in the last 10 years."
>
> *Therapist:* Mm-hmm, why do you think he keeps packing his suitcase?
>
> *Caregiver:* Well, I don't know, sometimes I think he wants to upset me. I can't explain it otherwise. He must see how much work it is for me.
>
> *Therapist:* And how do you feel when you think that he wants to upset you?
>
> *Caregiver:* It makes me furious. I have enough to do with him all day, so I don't need this as well.
>
> *Therapist:* Okay, it makes you angry, understandable, if you assume that he wants to upset you. Could there be other reasons besides his wanting to upset you?
>
> *Caregiver:* Mm-hmm, well he's pretty convinced that he's going on a journey. Perhaps he thinks it's like it was in the past, that he really is going on a journey.
>
> *Therapist:* Okay, did he used to travel a lot?
>
> *Caregiver:* Yes, on business, not so much personally, but he traveled a lot because of his company.
>
> *Therapist:* Yes, that sounds very plausible. Could it be that because of his illness, which doesn't allow him to orientate himself in time anymore, that he's convinced these days that he's going to travel again?
>
> *Caregiver:* Yes, that could very well be.
>
> *Therapist:* And if you look at it this way, how do you feel?
>
> *Caregiver:* [sigh] It makes it more understandable, why he keeps doing it, but it's still a burden for me.
>
> *Therapist:* Okay, so to start with, you say that it's more understandable.
>
> *Caregiver:* Yes.
>
> *Therapist:* Does that change your feeling?
>
> *Caregiver:* Yes, it makes me less angry. But I can't let him believe that he's going away.
>
> *Therapist:* It makes you less angry at first. The other thing is, you think you cannot let him believe that he's going on journey. Why not?
>
> *Caregiver:* Mm-hmm, I don't know. He's not going anywhere and then he'll surely be disappointed?
>
> *Therapist:* And he's not disappointed when you unpack his suitcase?
>
> *Caregiver:* No, of course he is, every time. Or rather, he's actually more upset. And that also exhausts me.
>
> *Therapist:* I understand. Could you maybe see it differently? So, you say that you can't let him believe that he's going away? Could a different thought provide you with relief in dealing with the situation?
>
> *Caregiver:* I could say to myself: "Let him do it, maybe he feels good doing it, like he used to. Then just leave the suitcase packed, it doesn't matter [laughs]."
>
> *Therapist:* How would you feel then?

Caregiver: Better, calmer.

Therapist: And your dad?

Caregiver: Well, he would probably feel more validated, maybe more useful or something like that.

Therapist: Yes, I find that a good thought. It would probably benefit his self-esteem, that he's still traveling.

Caregiver: Yes, you've given me a really good idea, I never saw it that way before.

Psychoeducation 5. Behavioral experiments (according to Stangier et al., 2003)

Many family caregivers have negative ideas about what other people could think about their person with dementia family member in public ("People will look at us strangely and talk about us"). These fears can be tested and changed in the context of a behavioral experiment. Behavioral experiments are a method of cognitive restructuring, in which the caregivers are instructed to reappraise negative expectations, irrational attitudes, or fears. The repeated experience that the expectations or fears do not occur in reality leads to the formation of new patterns of perception and interpretation (translated from German, Wittchen & Hoyer, 2006, p. 960).

9.2.6 Problem-Solving Strategies for Behavior Modification

After psychoeducation, behavioral analyses, and modification of dysfunctional appraisals have been completed, the next step is to consider and plan specific behavioral changes (see Case Example 20).

In doing so, it is important to respond individually to the situation and, based on the problem analyses, find solutions that are tailored to the family caregivers' needs. The information sheets presented can also be used to collect ideas. In order to empower the caregivers' experience of self-efficacy, it is important that caregivers search for solutions as independently as possible and that therapists provide ideas or solutions only as needed. Therapists can decide whether they merely dispute new

---

Case Example 20. Developing behavior modification with respect to accusations from the person with dementia (continuation of Case Example 18)

Therapist: Okay, we've already found out that yelling at your husband when he accuses you of having other men in bed doesn't help.

Caregiver: No, it just makes things worse.

Therapist: Okay, and what was your goal again?

Caregiver: That I can deal with it better, calmer. And that he then stops getting physically closer to me, I don't want that anymore.

Therapist: All right. Let's think about it: What could alternative approaches to your previous actions be? How else could you behave?

Caregiver: Mm-hmm, I could try to explain to him calmly that I've never cheated on him and that I will not do that anymore at my age.

Therapist: Mm-hmm, okay, you could try explaining that to him. How does that work in other situations when you try to explain something to him?

Caregiver: Well, actually, he doesn't understand much anymore. That doesn't really work anymore. I think sometimes that he's no longer able to understand what I mean.

Therapist: That means it might not work so well in this case also?

Caregiver: Yes, exactly. Probably not.

Therapist: Let's keep looking. What else can you think of?

Caregiver: I could just not react to it, ignore it.

Therapist: If you imagine that now. Your husband says to you "You have other men in your bed again!" How does it feel in your imagination to ignore that?

Caregiver: Not bad at all, actually, but he still wouldn't stop.

Therapist: Ok, what else is needed?

Caregiver: I would probably have to leave the room. Just go out. Maybe say: "I forgot something downstairs" or something like that.

Therapist: Yes, I think that's a good idea. What do you think the consequences would be if you tried it this way?

Caregiver: I could imagine that he'll have forgotten about it when I get back to the bedroom.

Therapist: Yes, that could be. How would you feel with this version?

Caregiver: Better, because then I wouldn't have a guilty conscience afterward, as if I would yell at him every time.

Therapist: Okay, so you would feel better?

Caregiver: Yes, absolutely.

Therapist: Good, would you like to try it out next time?

Caregiver: Yes, I'll try, to just go out and gain time. But he may still want to get physically close to me. This is often the case in the evenings when we go to bed.

Therapist: Yes, that's an additional problem. Let's think about how you could handle it. You said that you don't want that anymore?

Caregiver: No. Well, it's okay to hold his hand or to hug him and I also find it nice when he hugs me, but I don't want more.

Therapist: Do you have an idea what could help you in that situation?

Caregiver: Well, in this case I can't leave the bedroom every time. I still have to sleep somewhere.

Therapist: Okay. And you want to keep sleeping in a bed with him?

Caregiver: Well, I could also imagine sleeping alone. But, I don't know …

Therapist: Would that be possible?

Caregiver: Yes, we have a big house. I also move to the guest room every now and then when he snores.

Therapist: So, the possibility exists and you've already had experience with it?

Caregiver: Yes, actually.

Therapist: Okay. But it's still not the right solution?

Caregiver: Well, I would probably just need to take the plunge. It would be the best. I would feel safer, even if that sounds strange.

Therapist: You would feel safer?

Caregiver: Yes, and then the next morning I would probably be happier to see him because I will have slept better and not have had to reject him.

Therapist: Okay, could you imagine doing that in the future?

Caregiver: Yes, I'll give it a try.

Therapist: As a kind of experiment to test how you then feel?

Caregiver: Yes, I can imagine doing that.

solutions or use classical problem-solving training, according to D'Zurilla and Goldfried (1971, as described in Chapter 11).

For both intervention possibilities, these steps can be utilized as a guideline:
- problem definition and formulation;
- brief description of the goals set;
- collecting possible solutions;
- evaluating the possible solutions;
- planning and implementation of the possible solutions; and
- evaluation.

Case Example 21 focuses on the difficult situation of how to cope with delusional symptoms and intense anxiety of the person with dementia. It will become clear that there are generally no simple solutions to this challenging situation, but that in a longer process various options and creative ideas have to be found and tried out in everyday life. Furthermore, it will become apparent that trying to understand the anxiety of the person with dementia has a relieving effect on the caregivers and is a prerequisite for finding constructive solutions.

When developing new solutions and behaviors, it is important to convey the experimental character and work continuously on further adjustment and improvement. In my experience, it has proven to be supportive to assist caregivers in helping themselves and to recommend possibilities where they can obtain information, for example, from Alzheimer's association telephone services or local Alzheimer's association counseling centers, in order to be able to solve problems independently after counseling.

> **Case Example 21. Psychoeducation and problem solving for delusional symptoms and anxiety (continuation of Case Example 17)**
>
> *Caregiver:* It's usually the case that she shouts "Mom!" when I've brought her to bed in the evening. Then once I've sat down in the living room, she's like a broken record, and so loud. "MOM!" – "You promised me to be quiet. I'm right next door and you're here in bed, please be quiet!" But I don't succeed. I don't know. ... You can't do anything to calm her down when she's in this delusion and has a crying fit.
>
> *Therapist:* Exactly, it's a delusion. She's really imagining that she's freezing or drowning.
>
> *Caregiver:* Or that animals are biting her. That is also one of her fears.
>
> *Therapist:* It is difficult, I think, to convince her of the contrary, because that's not her reality and not the world in which she is at this moment. What you already tried to do during the day, that you say you get rid of the snakes or take them away ...
>
> *Caregiver:* Yes, I did that with her. But, how should I take away a lion?
>
> *Therapist:* Maybe you can react to your mother's imagination and say that you're going to take the lion outside. So, to play with her images. She will not believe that there's no lion, because she sees the lion. In other words, maybe it will calm her if you say: "I'm taking the lion outside now" or "With sedatives or sleeping pills, the lion is sleeping now and I'm taking him away." Or when she says that she's freezing: Instead of saying "You're not cold at all" – after all, that's what she perceives at the moment – you could say: "I'm going to cover you up so that you can get warm again." So that you can try to look at things from her perspective.
>
> *Caregiver:* There is the information sheet "anxiety" here. And they write here under Misjudgment and Hallucinations, "Chase away the frightening beings."
>
> *Therapist:* Yes, for some it helps to really say: "Now I'm chasing the snake away and I'm taking the lion outside."
>
> *Caregiver:* Yes, I already did that. I said: "Look, there's no snake here, and if there is one here, then I'll catch it and put it away."
>
> *Therapist:* Exactly, once you said that it worked out just fine when you told her, that you took the snakes and threw them into the lake near you. She was able to understand what you said and was calmed down for a moment. It's an attempt. One has to try it out.

9.2.7 Accepting Feelings Related to Challenging Behavior

Challenging behavior can also induce feelings of anxiety and disgust in many caregivers (Example 14).

Example 14. Fearing the person with dementia

> *Caregiver:* I'm afraid at night. We have been sleeping separately for a long time, but I am afraid that the door will open and that he will be standing in the door frame. It's already happened. I have nightmares often. I lock the door at night, I'm also afraid of body contact and closeness.

The first step is to analyze to what extent the fears are appropriate and realistic for the specific situation and to examine, in detail, how the situations have occurred so far. Furthermore, possible triggers for the person with dementia's threatening behavior are to be identified and possible modifications discussed. Helpful behavioral modifications and solution strategies are then to be derived according to the procedure described in Section 9.2.6.

If the caregiver cannot effectively influence the triggers and the problematic behavior in everyday care, other ways have to be found. In the event of a real threat and physically aggressive behavior of the person with dementia, which cannot be influenced by modifying the caregivers' behavior, medication of the symptoms or, if necessary, a change in the care situation should be considered (additional/other caregiver, professionally or familial; institutional care).

Family caregivers sometimes experience disgust due to certain behavioral or somatic symptoms of the person with dementia (see Case Example 22). Typical triggers of disgust are excrement and dirtiness. Disgust arises also when caregivers feel obliged to do something that they do not want to do or that violates their values.

Feelings of disgust often go hand in hand with feelings of helplessness, shame, and anger. It is important to care-

Case Example 22. Feelings of disgust

The following excerpt stems from therapy with a 65-year-old caregiving daughter.

Caregiver: I always have to wash everything. There is no other way. There is the bathroom rug and the tiles – everything is full in the bathroom. Last Friday I had to go to town. I asked him beforehand: "Do you have to go to the bathroom again, father?" – "No, no." I was only gone for 20 minutes at the most. When I came back, he was already standing at the door and said: "I heard you." Then I said: "What does it smell like here? Did you go to the bathroom?" – "No, no," he said. Oh ... the bathroom looked terrible. I was furious. I was beside myself! And I had even asked him before I went into town. I don't know if he's doing it deliberately, if he wants to mess with me. I don't know.

Therapist: What do you think?

Caregiver: I always think that he has to notice it. Nobody can tell me that he doesn't notice. It's not liquid. If it were liquid and he would really have diarrhea – that's all to be forgiven. I would see that. But this sticks to his behind. You can see that it has been there for a longer time.

Therapist: So, you think he should have noticed?

Caregiver: Yes, I would say so. I don't know. In the care facility, he *does not* do that!

Therapist: Dealing with stool incontinence really is one of the greatest challenges in caregiving. I hear from many family caregivers how burdensome and exhausting it is. And it is very understandable that you say: "This is my limit, I need some time, distance, or someone to help me with it."

Caregiver: Right, that's actually the case. I always say that if it's from a child, it's completely different than from an adult.

Therapist: Yes, absolutely.

Caregiver: That's just how it is. Nobody can tell me otherwise. Well [exhales deeply], nevertheless I'm relieved now that you suggested getting professional help. I know that I will do that. I'm sure.

fully analyze with the caregivers which appraisals and interpretations of the challenging behaviors trigger the feelings of disgust and which alternatives in behavior are possible. The personal boundaries of the caregivers should be made clear and respected and the use of external support services (e.g., nursing services) should be discussed.

In addition, family caregivers can be supported in verbalizing their feelings and burdensome thoughts (e.g., "Are you embarrassed when your husband constantly speaks to strangers?"). Validating thoughts and emotions in difficult situations ("I can understand that you react irritably in such situations") and normalizing these ("Many relatives report disgust in such situations") provide great relief for the caregivers (see also Chapter 10).

Especially for anxiety and disgust, it is particularly important to consider the limits of therapeutic work with family caregivers. It is not always possible to find constructive solutions for these extreme situations. In addition, the individual breaking points are very different and must be considered when finding a solution.

Additional therapeutic recommendations for dealing with burdensome feelings are given in Chapter 10 and Chapter 12.

10 "Anger Is Completely Normal" – Stress Management and Emotion Regulation

It is not only the person with dementia who often experience burdensome emotional states such as anxiety, restlessness, dejection, anger, frustration, and aggressiveness (see Example 15). Family caregivers also react to the extremely demanding caregiving situation with burdensome and unwanted impulses and emotions, especially rage, anger, and sometimes also unintentional aggressive actions. As a consequence of these feelings, especially when they are expressed as aggression toward the dementia sufferer, family caregivers experience massive feelings of shame and guilt. The subsequent feelings of self-reproach lead to an increased experience of burden and can set a vicious cycle in motion, which can result in developing depressive symptoms and anxiety regarding one's own impulsiveness as well as insecurity with respect to caregiving competence. In the long term, this can also compromise the caregivers' self-esteem.

Example 15. Feelings of anger and experiencing loss of control

> *Caregiver:* At that moment, yes, I'll say it, *hate* appears. So, on the really bad days, I say: "My God, you could *shake* him now so that he can think clearly again." It probably *wouldn't* be difficult for me to do that.
>
> *Therapist:* On those days where you feel so much hate, right?
>
> *Caregiver:* Yes, exactly. I feel rage, I'll honestly admit that. Because nobody can tell me that you can just stomach such things.

Many family caregivers find it difficult to admit their anger toward the person with dementia. This can be due to their lack of awareness of their feelings, to their not wanting to "bad-mouth" the person with dementia since they have already been "punished" enough by the illness. Moreover, admitting their anger may not reflect one's own personal ideals regarding caregiving and/or societal or internalized norms and values. In addition to the excessive demands, the sources of anger are often thoughts related to being left alone by the person with dementia with many worries and hardships, or thoughts related to the fact that previous conflicts can no longer be resolved. This can be the case, for example, if family caregivers had desired different behavior or more love from the person with dementia and had experienced the mutual relationship rather unhappily. The changed situation with the dementia sufferer's illness can lead to the caregiver feeling obligated to "have to" take care of them while simultaneously feeling angry about never having gotten what they had wanted from them.

In summary, family caregivers are often confronted with the following mutually dependent emotional states:
- fury, anger, aggressiveness;
- feelings of shame and guilt; and
- depressiveness, anxieties, and uncertainty.

This chapter focuses on acute burdensome situations in which feelings of fury and anger usually predominate. Therefore, the following sections focus on intervention suggestions for dealing with these emotions. The other emotions mentioned above are considered to be consequences which are discussed in further chapters of this manual: Coping with feelings related to the constant changes in life as a result of the illness, such as grief, guilt, and fear of the future, are addressed in Chapter 12, and dealing with feelings of shame is discussed in Chapter 9.

10.1 Goals of the Module

Family caregivers experience fury and anger on the one hand due to their inability to meet their self-imposed, usually too highly set, perfectionist demands regarding caregiving and dealing with their ill family member. On the other hand, caregivers experience these emotions, because the dementia sufferer's problem behavior and secondary symptoms can be extremely strenuous and demanding (see Chapter 9). In these acutely stressful situations, family caregivers often fail to react calmly and to classify and accept the dementia sufferer's behavior as symptomology of the illness. These stressful emotional states usually have easily comprehensible causes, which can be worked out with the caregivers in the therapeutic sessions.

Box 13 contains an overview of the interventions regarding the different subjects covered in this chapter.

Box 13. Overview of the interventions

1. decatastrophizing emotions such as fury and anger and accepting and understanding them as normal reactions to an extraordinary stressful situation;
2. finding short-term possibilities to distance oneself from burdensome feelings in order to cool down and then be able to analyze the situation;
3. determining, reviewing, and applying adequate options for action;
4. developing ways of expressing and regulating feelings;
5. promoting acceptance of challenging behavior and the occurrence of undesirable feelings, especially if the person with dementia's behavior is recurring and not changeable; and
6. working on the general level of tension.

10.2 Therapeutic Approach

The therapeutic approach is divided into several substeps and includes different intervention methods such as knowledge transfer, problem analysis, problem solving, cognitive restructuring, stress management techniques, and techniques for emotion regulation. In this chapter, techniques for stress management and emotion regulation in particular are explained. As a general rule, the use of other CBT strategies for coping with acute stress are also helpful and necessary.

Case Example 23 illustrates how the goals and usefulness of a strategy for reducing stress responses in problematic situations can be imparted.

10.2.1 Decatastrophizing and Normalization of Fury and Anger in Acute Stress Situations

Family caregivers experience it as a great relief when they learn that other family caregivers experience similar impulses and emotions. Clarifying that it is normal and human to react with negative feelings in challenging, stressful situations usually has an immediate relieving effect on family caregivers (Psychoeducation 6).

Case Example 23. Explanation of the goals

The following excerpt stems from therapy with a 78-year-old caregiving husband.

Caregiver: Yes, neglect, but also feelings of hate. Feelings arise that make me want to beat her, sometimes.

Therapist: Maybe we can write that down as a goal that you want to gain a little more emotional distance, okay?

Caregiver: Correct. Exactly. Yes, maybe ... how should I put it now, so ... well, I don't want to end up facing the whole thing with indifference or professionalism.

Therapist: Yes. I understand.

Caregiver: I don't want to be like nursing staff, who don't let anything get to them anymore. Actually, it comes with the territory that it burdens and affects you.

Therapist: Yes, of course. It's a relationship.

Caregiver: But it shouldn't be that I'm in such despair because of this.

Therapist: Perhaps we can describe it in such a way that you want a balance ... that you are emotionally there for your wife and can be reached, but that it doesn't turn into despair.

Caregiver: Yes, exactly. So, I would say a balance between feeling and handling it rationally.

Therapist: Yes. So, a balance between experiencing your emotions and being able to distance yourself at the right moment. For such stressful and emotional situations, I would like to introduce you to procedures that can help you to perceive and control physical and emotional excitement in these situations, to reduce stress and to act deliberately.

Psychoeducation 6. Normalizing fury

Therapist: What we know from talks with family caregivers is that sometimes things can accumulate, leading to even more anger and unpleasant feelings and all it takes is one thing to be the last straw. And that's why it makes sense to continuously reduce the anger.

Caregiver: Yes, I think so too. I can already imagine that if I can't deflate this anger, it will make itself noticeable in my body at some point and I will probably explode in a situation where it's not appropriate. Because then I'm irritated, right?

Therapist: Well, when it comes to such stressors, it is understandable that you reach a point where you say: "I am totally irritated now, so much that I would like to isolate myself or start bawling." You just get very thin-skinned when you're constantly stressed.

In this context it is also important to address taboo topics such as aggressive actions toward the person with dementia (see Case Example 24). Therapists should acknowledge the high level of stress that sometimes arises when dealing with the person with dementia, and also validate behaviors that are not always helpful, such as aggressive counter-behavior or insults. This usually allows family members to speak for the first time about their culpable thoughts and actions, and to learn to process and change them.

While violence in caregiving should be openly addressed, this does not mean that the topic should be left as it is and viewed as an irreversible consequence. On the contrary, family caregivers are given the opportunity to speak about such incidences so that they can learn how to change their behavior and reflect on how such actions (verbal or physical) can be prevented in the future.

In the next step, the therapist and family caregivers consider together which behaviors can lead to an improvement of the respective situation and a reduction of stressful emotions (Case Example 25). Moreover, systematic

Case Example 24. Addressing taboo topics

The following excerpt stems from therapy with a 78-year-old caregiving wife.

Caregiver: I've always said: "I can do anything, but if he gets aggressive, then I don't know how I'll act."

Therapist: Mm-hmm, I understand.

Caregiver: Well, it takes a lot of my strength; I really have to control myself, very much [crying].

Therapist: Yes, I can understand that very well. It's really difficult.

Caregiver: I mean, I have dealt with his fantasies and also with him soiling his pants. That didn't bother me. But this reluctance and those ... vulgar expressions sometimes, you know? It's awful.

Therapist: Yes, I understand that well.

Caregiver: And to be completely honest ... I'm ashamed of it now ... but there are moments ... I can't control myself ... I just can't.

Therapist: Yes, and what happens then?

Caregiver: [Crying] I scream at him.

Therapist: Yes, his behavior makes you furious.

Caregiver: Yes, but then I have to be calm, I have to be calm, I am not allowed to do that, otherwise I will get worked up even more. Then I think: "You have to swallow it all quickly, you mustn't be like that."

Therapist: Yes, you don't want that ... that's okay too, but I think the rage you feel is a perfectly normal reaction to the situation.

Caregiver: No, you know, I have to remove myself from the situation then, otherwise ... dear God ... I don't know what else will happen one day.

Therapist: I think leaving the situation is a good idea, but at the same time it is important to acknowledge that the anger you are feeling is actually a normal feeling.

Caregiver: Yes, but I'm just afraid that I'll no longer be able to control myself ... that's the problem and I can't let that happen, no way.

> **Case Example 25. Accepting fury and anger**
>
> The following excerpt stems from therapy with a 43-year-old caregiving daughter.
>
> *Therapist:* What does that mean for you that you realize that she has forgotten it again?
>
> *Caregiver:* For me, it means that I'm actually upset about something that makes no sense.
>
> *Therapist:* That you get upset about something that doesn't make sense. Why does it make no sense?
>
> *Caregiver:* Because I notice that she doesn't even know what she was talking about. And I also know that she didn't mean it that way, could not have meant it that way. And then I automatically feel insulted until I notice that I shouldn't feel that way.
>
> *Therapist:* It's legitimate that you feel insulted and get upset, and the agitation is allowed to find an outlet. The thing is, your mother is not the right outlet, because you say: "I notice that she has forgotten it again," but that means, so to speak, that your agitation still means something, specifically, that you experienced an insult that you have to deal with. And it is understandable that you feel insulted. That doesn't mean that you should "shoot back" at your mother, but it does make sense to admit fury and anger and to allow it: "That is allowed to be there."

instructions for dealing with acutely burdensome emotions are given.

10.2.2 Dealing With Strong Emotionality: Four Steps for Dealing With Acute Stressful Situations

This therapeutic intervention was taken from the manual by Kaluza (2015, pp. 185–189) and modified for working with family caregivers. The therapist explains to the family caregivers that the procedure consists of a total of four steps and should help them in acute stressful situations to be able to keep calm and be capable of acting reasonably. During the explanations, the family caregivers are provided with Worksheet 10-1: Short Exercise for Coping With Acute Stress.

As the first step, *understanding* is addressed with the family caregivers (see Psychoeducation 7).

Psychoeducation 7. Understanding and accepting burden

> *Therapist:* The first step is *understanding* the burden (for example, the person with dementia's problem behavior). This means accepting the situation (the behavior) as it is – as a part of dementia, as part of your everyday caregiving routine. Anger, accusations, and feelings of guilt help just as little as not wanting it to be true.
>
> Accepting the situation involves two different things:
> 1. detecting signals that indicate a difficult situation as early as possible; and
> 2. a clear and conscious decision to accept the difficult situation (and thus not fighting against reality).
>
> If you notice that you are feeling annoyed and furious, then allow it to be that way. This really is the very first step in order to understand what's going on with you. That is just how it is at that given moment. And now you can take out the worksheet for the short exercise for coping with acute stress out of the folder.
>
> *Caregiver:* "Short exercise for coping with acute stress."
>
> *Therapist:* Exactly, and what we just discussed is the very first point: acceptance. Also accepting *yourself*. You have described that your father does not respond to you with aggression, but that he acts toward you as he has always acted toward you, very nicely, right?
>
> *Caregiver:* Hmm, yes.
>
> *Therapist:* But you notice with yourself that it's simply a great burden, all of it together, that is, your own health, your own job, your husband at home, and you taking care of your father, which is altogether a lot. And then you get into a situation that you may have already experienced a thousand times, to the point that you realize: "Wow, now I'm getting into a rage."
>
> *Caregiver:* Hmm, yes.
>
> *Therapist:* That's okay to notice that for now. So maybe it's helpful in the situation to then *label* it for yourself. As if you were looking at yourself from the outside and say-

ing: "Okay, I can now see that this makes me angry." And it's helpful to tell yourself that mentally too.

Caregiver: Yes, yes.

Therapist: Because you realize that you are *not* your feelings, but that you *have* these feelings. They are just a part of you and you can observe them, but you are *not* your feelings, and, yes, there are other things too. Feelings come and feelings go, and it's something that comes, and that is okay that it comes, and then it goes again, okay? And then allow yourself to pause for a moment.

In the next step, possibilities for distancing oneself from the acute feelings are discussed in order to then be able to analyze the situation more clearly and gauge coping strategies. Helpful distancing techniques are developed with the caregivers individually and specific options for "cooling down" in an acute problem situation are sought after.

The caregivers are asked to write down an individual possible way for them to cool down on Worksheet 10-1: Short Exercise for Coping With Acute Stress (see Psychoeducation 8).

Psychoeducation 8. Cooling down

Therapist: The second step is *cooling down*. This means getting a grip on your own strong agitation when you are "beside yourself," "wanting to go through the roof," or "losing your composure." It's about composing yourself, grounding yourself, and keeping a clear head. How can this be done? By consciously choosing to cool down and deciding against getting all worked up about the agitation. Cooling off can happen by consciously extending your exhalation, with which the "steam" is released. But you can also try to relax consciously or do short movement exercises.

Do you already have strategies for yourself that you can do in order to slow down a bit inside?

Caregiver: Yes, so sometimes I leave the room. It's mostly in the bathroom when he ... and then I often go out and let him sit for a while.

Therapist: How do you feel about it when you go out?

Caregiver: Yes, I'm a little calmer then.

In Psychoeducation 9, the acute problem situation is analyzed with respect to the question of whether it can be changed through action or whether there are no possibilities for change. In order to be capable of analyzing the situation, it needs to be recapitulated that the previously discussed inner distance is needed in order to make this decision. Should the caregivers recognize possible courses of action after the short problem analysis, constructive possible solutions are then developed by using problem-solving training.

Psychoeducation 9. Analyzing

Therapist: The third step is *analyzing* the problem situation, i.e., taking a moment to come to a conscious evaluation of the situation. You can do this by asking yourself: "Can I do/change something right now?" If so, you can take *action*, for example, by calling an emergency doctor, seeking support, rescheduling appointments, rearranging care tasks, etc.

Afterward, options for "actions" (possible solutions) for the specific problem situation are sought after and assessed with the caregivers (e.g., Psychoeducation 10). Detailed examples for the development for specific solutions are also presented in Chapter 9.

Psychoeducation 10. Distraction

Therapist: If you find that there is nothing you can do/change right now, then try *distracting* yourself, for example, by retreating, listening to music, thinking about something pleasant, or calling someone, etc.

Moreover, further individually suitable strategies on how to distance oneself from fury or anger are sought after and discussed with the caregivers. Box 14 provides a few examples of ways to distance oneself.

Box 14. Examples of techniques for distancing oneself (according to Lammers, 2011, p. 238)

- Turn around and walk away
- Corrective self-instructions (e.g., "Stop!" or "Do not respond any further!")
- Positive self-verbalizations (e.g., "I am strong and controlled.")
- Count to 100
- Consciously concentrated breathing
- Thought stopping

In addition to the techniques of distancing and distracting oneself from burdening emotions, direct expression of the feelings can be of essential importance for psychological well-being (see also Chapter 12). However, many caregivers do not know how to deal with these feelings. Therefore, in the therapeutic sessions, ways that help in reducing tension and venting the feelings of anger are sought after. Crying, screaming, or physical exercise are possibilities for relieving tension and can be necessary for managing stress and dealing with the burden. Another example is illustrated by a family caregiver who bought a trampoline. Whenever the caregiving situation was too stirring and impended to escalate, the caregiver went to the adjoining room to jump on the trampoline. Several caregivers also exercise or work out in nature to reduce tension (see Case Example 26).

It should be noted, however, that this "acting out" should not occur in the presence of people with dementia, as they are usually overwhelmed by strong negative emotions from the people present and can in turn react with burdensome reactions and emotions.

10.2.3 Encouragement of Understanding and Acceptance

Especially when the person with dementia's challenging behavior is recurring and difficult to change, accepting one's own undesirable feelings can be meaningful.

The utilization of strategies from acceptance and commitment therapy (e.g., Luoma et al., 2008) offers a supportive perspective in this context. Acceptance here means to perceive and experience negative and stressful feelings, thoughts, and sensations without directly changing or avoiding them (Case Example 27).

Another possibility to encourage an accepting attitude regarding one's own emotionality is to ask the caregivers to bring to mind what is going on internally in the situation. In the mindfulness literature this is referred to as "informal mindfulness practice" (cf. Meibert et al., 2010) with the goal of promoting sensitivity for one's own mental state. In moments of emotional activation, the caregivers should change into this practiced attitude, for example: "I am just noticing that I am tense and that I am starting to get angry." The verbalization of the emotional experience enables a behavior modification by creating and enabling a certain internal and also temporal distance to one's own emotionality. Then, the caregivers do not fall into automated, "familiar" behaviors, but there is the possibility of applying newly learned behavior.

In addition, small mindfulness exercises can be practiced with the caregivers (see Box 15).

Case Example 26. Venting stressful feelings of fury

The following excerpt stems from therapy with a 63-year-old caregiving wife.

Therapist: You say you manage to calm down pretty well, for example, by having a cup of coffee or cleaning up. Is there an exercise about which you say: "I can really let off steam?"

Caregiver: Yes, for example I can go into the garden and chop wood.

Therapist: Okay, that's a good idea. Have you done that before?

Caregiver: I've done that before [laughs briefly].

Therapist: Okay.

Caregiver: Yes, it works, it works … so far somehow.

Therapist: So, you have already tried that out. Immediately after an insulting situation, you went into the garden to chop wood. Great. And even if it is just one log.

Caregiver: Yes, exactly, so that I can blow off some steam.

Therapist: And it also doesn't take too much time?

Caregiver: Exactly!

Therapist: The idea of dealing with feeling hurt or the agitation, tension, anger, by chopping wood or pulling weeds or sweeping the courtyard, in order to blow off a little bit of steam, I think that's absolutely great.

Case Example 27. Encouraging acceptance of burdensome feelings

The following excerpt stems from therapy with a 77-year-old caregiving wife.

Caregiver: I think that's what makes me so unhappy: I would like to be mellow and kind, but I have this feeling of rage in my gut.

Therapist: Exactly. And if you judge yourself for having this rage in your gut …

Caregiver: … I get sadder and sadder.

Therapist: You get sadder and sadder and you can't be happy either.

Caregiver: Mm-hmm [crying].

Therapist: That does not work. That contradicts itself.

Caregiver: Yes [crying]. You wouldn't believe how much literature there is, strangely enough, from men who care for their sick wife with devoted love.

Therapist: Of course there are people who do that. I think what is important for you to know is that it doesn't have to work that way. You don't have to get absorbed in the care, you don't have to say: "I don't care about anything else. I'll do without what's important to me in life." You don't have to give all of that up.

Caregiver: So, I can just stand by my feelings and say: "I don't have to change my feelings."

Therapist: Yes. That is what I'd like to tell you.

Caregiver: Yes, yes.

Therapist: That is the first step. To accept that these feelings are there and that feelings are something very important. They show us the way in life. And pushing them away makes them become worse and worse, and leads to you reacting to caregiving in a way that you actually don't want.

Caregiver: Yes.

Therapist: And so, it would be an important task for you starting now to start paying much more attention to how you're feeling in the moment and to calmly allow these feelings to occur.

That you, when you are with your husband, consider which behavior is useful for the situation, which is most useful for both of you, which is gentler for both of you. But the most important thing is that those feelings that you still have at this moment are okay.

Caregiver: That they are okay.

Therapist: Yes.

Caregiver: That was always the problem, because I felt so mean. I felt so insincere. I have to separate it more clearly now. That it's okay to have the feelings but that it's also necessary to handle the situation reasonably.

Box 15. The 5–4–3–2–1 exercise (Bambach, 2006, pp. 248–253)

The aim of the exercise is to anchor yourself in the present, in order to be able to detach yourself from strong emotions.

Take a comfortable sitting position in your chair.

As a start I would like to ask you to concentrate on 5 things that you can see at this moment. List (in your mind) 5 things that you can see right now. Next, I ask you to perceive 5 things that you can hear. List (in your head) 5 things that you can hear.

And finally, I ask you to perceive 5 things that you can feel. List (in your head) 5 things that you can feel.

4 things that you see/hear/feel

3 things that you see/hear/feel

2 things that you see/hear/feel

1 thing that you see/hear/feel

Remain seated for a moment and observe the effect of the exercise on your body and on your mind. Generally, your hands get warm because the muscles relax and blood flow increases.

Caregiving family members experience it as an enormous relief to talk about these unwanted feelings and to find out that they can be understood empathetically. Above all, the information that several family caregivers feel similarly (best formulated as an exemplary narrative of a report from another family caregiver) and that these reactions are always an important topic in the therapy sessions, represents for the caregivers a meaningful and soothing, mostly unexpected experience (see Example 16).

Example 16. Evaluation of the intervention from a caregiving wife

> *Therapist:* Yes, Mrs. G., how are you feeling now at the end of our talk?
>
> *Caregiver:* Oh yeah, good.
>
> *Therapist:* What are you taking with you?
>
> *Caregiver:* That I can be angry [laughs slightly]. That I don't have to be ashamed of it. That I can get angry too.
>
> *Therapist:* Exactly, absolutely. So, I think that's something very important, to give yourself permission: "It's okay that I'm angry now."
>
> *Caregiver:* Yes, I'll take that with me now as a message. So, this has given me a lot now.

Additionally, in these interventions, the focus should be resource oriented and especially on the positive moments with the person with dementia. A relationship is seldom exclusively negative. However, if only negative aspects are remembered or discussed, this can make it even more difficult to adapt to the changes.

10.2.4 Work on the General Level of Tension

In principle, the work on acutely burdensome emotions can be supplemented by the additional intervention shown in Psychoeducation 11. By reducing the general level of tension, the overall likelihood of impulsive reactions and strong feelings of anger and fury can be reduced. In the context of this chapter, the dialogue in Psychoeducation 11 illustrates how psychoeducation on the meaning of the level of tension can be presented.

Psychoeducation 11. Work on level of tension

The following excerpt stems from therapy with a 66-year-old caregiving wife.

Therapist: In the situation that you described at the beginning of our talk, you mentioned that you were relaxed. You didn't have to get away from your husband at a certain time point, you had enough time and could relax into the situation. And that had a positive effect overall: You didn't show any anger, so there was no reason for him to react to your anger with his own anger. So, this had a positive effect in that the vicious cycle of anger was broken so to speak, and the situation was peaceful for both you and your husband. And that actually has something to do with the level of tension in the situation.

Caregiver: Yes, there is just often a certain amount of tension there.

Therapist: Exactly, so let's say you're already going into the situation with a level of tension – I'll just say a number, I don't know if it's true for you – 60/70%. You've had a very stressful day at work. So, you already have a relatively high level of tension with which you enter the situation. And if something happens there, of course – be it that you get strange advice or the milk is boiling over [jokingly] or whatever – then you can go from 60 to 80 faster, for example, than if you were at 30 going into the situation, as was the case now on vacation. If the milk boils over or your husband tells you something, you are at 50. Still, you can deal with the anger well at 50. When you hit 80 of course, it's difficult. You have reached the threshold, so to speak, and then it is clear that you are more irritable, end up in a rage or even start to cry.

Caregiver: Yes [laughs shortly].

Therapist: I'm sure you know a lot of examples. If you've had a strenuous day, then it adds up, then all you need is one little thing to be the last straw. So, I would like to gather ideas with you now: What can you do to reduce your level of tension? What can you do during the situation if it becomes difficult and you notice: "Now the tension is increasing, now the anger is rising, now I'm about to burst ..." – What can you do then in the situation to help you to defuse? And what is perhaps also important afterward – regardless of how the situation turned out, whether you were able to cope with it well or whether it turned out that the anger took off. What is important after that? This is how I would split it up: before, during, after. And we can consider now what would be important after the situation, so that you don't end up ruminating, getting into a spiral of feelings of guilt. Then we can consider what pleasant things you could do for yourself, for your well-being.

The caregivers can also be asked about their current level of tension in each session in order to sensitize them to their own perception. In addition, behavior and situation analyses can be used to inquire about the general level of tension in a situation, and to discuss with the caregivers which strategies can be used in the event of a high level of tension, for example, leaving the room, going for a walk. The objective of the promotion of self-care is linked to this topic and is presented in detail in Chapter 11.

11 "And What About Me?" – Self-Care and Value-Based Activities

Due to strong time constraints, the seldomly utilized professional support, existing dysfunctional thoughts and schemas (e.g., "I can't do something nice for myself while my husband is suffering so much at home," "It's a given that one is completely and utterly there for the other person") and the feelings associated with them (e.g., guilty conscience), there is a lack of self-care and balancing activities among most caregivers.

Exemplary statements on "lack of self-care and balancing activities"

- "I always say: 'I don't live at all anymore.' That I undertake something or do something for myself doesn't happen anymore. I want to live spontaneously, as I used to, visit a friend for an hour or half an hour. I can't do any of that anymore. I am very limited in my activities."
- "I don't get out of here anymore, sometimes I feel like I'm locked in. And he just sleeps all day. I can't even talk with him. What is left for me? Sometimes I feel really depressed, everything is so monotonous."
- "I don't have a life of my own anymore. I'm busy with her all day, from morning to evening, and I can't leave here, because I can't leave her alone anymore."
- "It's kind of unfair, he didn't choose this either and then I always have a guilty conscience when I do something for myself."

A constant lack of self-care and balancing activities can lead to long-term loss of quality of life, deterioration in mood, and ultimately the development of symptoms of depression. This not only has consequences for the caregiver, but also for the entire family system. Therefore, improving self-care and scheduling pleasant, meaningful activities presents an important topic in therapy with family caregivers.

11.1 Goals of the Module

The first goal of the module is to help caregivers realize the importance of self-care-related and balancing activities for their own health and well-being and to facilitate a motivation for change.

Afterward, caregivers' existing possibilities for self-care and established pleasant activities can be discussed. Subsequently, the planning and implementation of new activities in everyday life can be prepared and reflected upon together with the caregivers. Other modules, such as dealing with dysfunctional thoughts (Chapter 8) or improving the utilization of professional support services (Chapter 13), can be used here as well. Further goals are the maintenance of self-care activities in the long term and the prevention of potential "relapses" into familiar dysfunctional behavior patterns. Box 16 contains an overview of the interventions covered in this chapter.

Box 16. Overview of the interventions

- Imparting and clarifying the importance and necessity of self-care and taking up balancing activities
- Collecting, selecting, and planning suitable possibilities for self-care and balancing activities
- Problem-solving training to support planning and implementation
- Reflecting on the implementation and maintenance of self-care and the planned pleasant activities
- Normalization and acceptance of feelings of guilt

11.2 Therapeutic Approach

11.2.1 Imparting and Working Out the Importance and Necessity of Self-Care and Taking Up Balancing Activities

The therapeutic challenge in promoting self-care and taking up pleasant activities for family caregivers is due to the fact that they are often much more limited in time and with regard to location, compared to other clients. Therefore, the argumentation against taking up self-care activities put forward by family caregivers should be taken seriously. Nevertheless, there is no question that ways must also be found for family caregivers to establish a certain level of self-care in order to maintain their own health.

Thus, it can be useful to begin by imparting to the family caregivers the importance of self-care and enjoyable activities without directly considering how an improvement might look in their specific case. For a better illustration, Figure 1, based on Hautzinger, 2000, p. 139) can be used.

Psychoeducation 12. Scale model (based on Hautzinger, 2000, p. 139)

> *Therapist:* Yes, exactly, I find it very important that you say: "My battery is empty, I'm noticing that now and I need to do something for myself." That is your right. You've done an amazing job for a very long time and, as you say, you cannot do that without taking care of yourself. You can't just always be there for others without keeping an eye on yourself.

In order to remain resilient in the long term – according to this scale model – pleasant and unpleasant, stressful and enjoyable events should be more or less balanced. In order to prevent mental and physical overload, it makes sense that we also plan something pleasant for ourselves in our weekly routine. Pleasant and value-based experiences can improve our mood and also act as a buffer for other stressful experiences. The improved mood can in turn have a positive effect on our patience and strength, which we need in order to be able to cope well with everyday challenges. Possible consequences from a lack of balancing activities and thus a deterioration of the caregivers' own health can then be discussed (see Case Example 28).

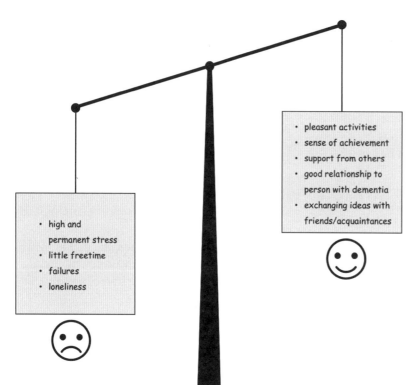

Figure 1. Scale model (based on Hautzinger, 2000)

Case Example 28. Consequences from a lack of balancing activities

The following case example stems from therapy with a 34-year-old caregiving daughter.

Caregiver: It's just difficult, to do more for myself, I simply don't have the time.

Therapist: Yes, you are short on time, that's right. We have already looked at the scale model and have seen that a balance with positive activities is very important. What do you think would happen if you continued like you have been for a few more months or even years?

Caregiver: I don't know, I would probably get more and more exhausted.

Therapist: And what would that mean?

Caregiver: That everything will be much more exhausting, maybe also ... that I will break down at some point. It already feels like that sometimes. But I really don't know how to change that, I have to be there for my father.

Therapist: You say that you might break down at some point.

Caregiver: Yes.

Therapist: What would that mean?

Caregiver: Hmm, everything would probably be too much for me then. I would no longer function.

Therapist: And what would be the consequences?

Caregiver: I could no longer be there for my family, would probably do nothing at all.

Therapist: Yes, that means you couldn't go on caring for your father either?

Caregiver: Nope, I couldn't do that then.

Therapist: Okay, that means, if you carry on as you do now, that is, you don't take enough care of yourself, because you always want to be there for your father, you might end up so exhausted one day that you can no longer take care of your father?

Caregiver: [laughs] That sounds kind of paradoxical now.

Therapist: Yes, I think so too. And what could you conclude from this?

Caregiver: Yes, probably that I have no other choice than to create more balance, because that's the only way I can care for him for a while longer.

Therapist: Yes, exactly, because taking care of your father is also important to you, right?

Caregiver: Yes, that is important to me. I can't imagine putting him in a home.

Therapist: Yes, I understand that. And how important is your health to you?

Caregiver: That is also very important to me.

Therapist: Could one say that both are important to you, but in order to be able to do one thing, you have to do the other first?

Caregiver: Yes, you could say that.

Working out the importance of one's own health and self-care is an important prerequisite for developing motivation to schedule pleasant activities. The caregivers can first be asked what they have done or what they have enjoyed in the past 7 days. It often becomes clear that the caregivers neglect their own needs in favor of the person with dementia. As a rule, family caregivers give many reasons why self-care-related behavior was not possible due to caregiving and why it will also be difficult to achieve in the future.

It can therefore make sense to first address the caregivers' personal values. Questions 12 are helpful in "tracking down" the caregivers' needs and values.

Questions 12. Exploring personal needs

> - What are important needs in your life?
> - What was previously important to you in your life (before the illness of your loved one)?
> - What gave you strength in the past?
> - In which direction should your life go?
> - What matters most in your life?
> - What should your life stand for?

For example, caregivers often neglect relationships or friendships due to caregiving (see Case Example 29). Using disputation techniques, therapists can determine with the caregivers which level of significance these areas of life have for them. Caregiving daughters, for instance, often state that their own relationship with their partner is more important than caring for a parent. However, caregivers usually do not act in accordance with their own needs, and it is not uncommon for caregiving children to give their own relationships or friendships less priority. It is important to point out this conflict of needs. In order to consider how a change in the sense of "more time with your partner or girlfriend" could occur, caregivers must first become aware that maintaining a good relationship with their partner or friends is also important to them. At the end of this phase, a hierarchy of values and needs can be drawn up with the caregivers and retained in written form.

Furthermore, caregivers often have dysfunctional thoughts with regard to the care receiver's well-being, for example fear that the person with dementia might feel very badly in the caregiver's absence or that the person with dementia might object to external care. In such cases, the application of cognitive restructuring methods is very helpful, for example by using the ABC model (see Case Example 13 and instructions in Chapter 8).

11.2.2 Promoting Self-Care: Collecting, Selecting, and Planning Balancing Activities

Strategies for scheduling activities and problem solving known from the treatment of depression can be helpful in promoting self-care and enjoyable activities.

After discussing the importance of self-care and balancing activities with the caregivers, questions can be asked about what self-care behavior looks like for them at the moment and what value-based and pleasant activities they are already doing. Therapists often discuss with the caregivers activities that they used to experience as pleasant but are no longer able to experience due to caregiving demands.

Sometimes the caregivers are so stressed over an extended period of time that they can no longer remember which activities would have a positive and relaxing effect. In Case Example 30, a family caregiver reports that his sense of his own needs has been lost.

Only when the caregiver has succeeded in creating some space and relieving some stress, their own needs and interests can be discussed again. Then it can be considered whether the caregiver has enough energy again to actively attend to interests and pleasant things and to in-

---

Case Example 29. Neglecting personal needs

The following excerpt stems from therapy with a 50-year-old caregiving daughter.

Therapist: So your marriage was also strained by the caregiving situation?

Caregiver: Very strained, very. My husband said, "Look, you have her in the home now. You need to stop thinking about it so much, and the stress, that you had before, cannot go on like this." I'm glad that he was so busy with his job. If I had had a husband who worked his eight hours every day and was home in the evenings and regularly on the weekends, my marriage would have run into a brick wall a long time ago.

Therapist: You think so?

Caregiver: Yes! I can assume so. No relationship can keep up with that, because no partner would tolerate that for so many years and do without free time and other pleasures together. The last time we were on vacation together was 5 years ago.

Therapist: Oh really?!

Case Example 30. Loss of awareness of one's own needs

The following excerpt stems from therapy with a 63-year-old caregiving husband.

Caregiver: In the past, I used to listen to music and use it to achieve or express certain moods. None of that works anymore. None of that reaches me anymore. It even annoys me already that have to choose a piece of music that I *might* be able to hear in the car – and then I don't do it. Sometimes, when I'm at a very low point, I say: "I, *me*, somehow no longer exist." To say, so to speak: "What do I like now, what could I hear now to relax?"

Therapist: Okay, you no longer have access to it, you don't know: "What do I need now?" – did I understand you correctly?

Caregiver: Yes.

Therapist: You are no longer really with yourself. That sounds like a lot of constant stress.

Caregiver: Yes, somehow I'm just functioning.

Therapist: That is also an important signal. That a limit has been reached here. "I'm just getting lost in the care." Could one see it like that?

Caregiver: Yes. It also makes me sad somehow that there is hardly any space left and that everything is too much for me, even listening to music is too much for me.

Therapist: I think it's important to take this seriously. A point has been reached where more space needs to be created for yourself and your needs. What do you think about that?

Caregiver: Yes, that's true …

Therapist: And that's not easy to do when you're so exhausted.

Caregiver: Yes, but even the thought of having to change something is also too much for me.

Therapist: It can be helpful to find the first small steps to relieve stress in your daily routine, and then to expand this over time. At your own pace. What could be a first small step here?

Caregiver: I would have to think about that.

Therapist: Perhaps it would help to think about: What tasks could I omit? Who could support me, take over something?

Case Example 31. Loss of awareness of one's own needs (continuation from Case Example 30)

Therapist: Well, I think that's a great idea with the music, and with that there's a starting point. It's more difficult if one says: "I have no idea what's good for me." But I don't think that's the case. You just have to reactivate it. And therefore, what would be a very concrete goal? That you said: "Until next week I'll look through a certain number of CDs or I will select a piece to try." What could you imagine that wouldn't completely overwhelm you but that you could really achieve?

Caregiver: Well, I could imagine to say: I'll select five CDs, perhaps five quite different types of music, and put them in my car, really put them on, and then see what happens there and how I feel when I hear them. Whether that annoys me again right away and I turn them off [laughs shortly] or … I don't know. But it would be an attempt.

Therapist: Okay, that would be something very specific. That you pick out five CDs and see if you notice that you are becoming more relaxed, get rid of stress, and think about something else. Would you imagine that you could do that?

tegrate them back into their everyday life. This topic is continued in the Case Example 31.

The Worksheets 11-2: Suggestions for Pleasant Activities (based on Hautzinger, 2000, p. 75 ff.) and 11-3: Suggestions for Self-Care can be used to help with identifying pleasant activities.

Then it should be discussed which pleasant activities and self-care behaviors the caregivers can imagine integrating into their everyday life in the future. In addition to specific actions, the attitude toward oneself is particularly important when promoting self-care. Then it can be agreed upon to try to eat healthier in the future, to look for opportunities to laugh, or to dress pleasantly. Generally, this makes it easier for caregivers to focus more on themselves than by planning specific activities. For this purpose, Worksheet 11-4: My Current Weekly Plan can be given as homework, on which the caregivers write down a typical week for them.

Once the information has been filled in, therapists can use disputation to work out which duties the caregivers can withdraw from or how their day can be divided more sensibly so that there is freedom to plan and incorporate pleasant activities. Then it can be considered which pleasant experiences can be integrated into the daily routine without additional planning or support measures, which pleasant activities the person with dementia can benefit from, and which activities can be carried out together without the need for an additional caregiver or an accompanying person.

Such activities, which are easier to implement, can be planned and discussed directly with the caregivers. A weekly plan (Worksheet 11-5: My New Weekly Plan) can be used to support this. Caregivers can fill in which activities they plan to undertake on which day and at which time, as well as activities for which they still need time to plan, if necessary.

Additionally, reminder aids should be created, for example with sticky notes or cards that can be hung up at home, or with reminders in their mobile phone or on the calendar.

11.2.3 Problem-Solving Training for Planning and Implementing Pleasant Activities

It is not uncommon for some activities, such as a trip or a visit to a theatre, to appear unfeasible at first, for example due to the unavailability of another caregiving person. Here an attempt can be made to find solutions using problem-solving training according to D'Zurilla and Goldfried (1971) (see Box 17 and Worksheet 11-6: Six Steps for Problem Solving).

Box 17. Problem-solving training according to D'Zurilla and Goldfried (1971)

1. Explaining the meaning and necessity of the problem-solving approach
2. Brief description of a problem or the jointly developed needs
3. Brief description of the goal setting
4. Collecting possible solutions ("brainstorming")
5. Evaluating the possible solutions
6. Planning and implementing possible solutions
7. Evaluate the result and possible run through the problem-solving process again

If the problem-solving training method yields possibilities for how caregivers can indeed undertake positive activities toward which they were initially doubtful, these activities can also be included in the weekly plan.

Therapeutic guidance: Planning and implementing self-care activities

Therapist: Ok, good. I notice that you're generally good at analyzing problems. You think, "What is the problem and how can I describe and solve it?" Exactly, and now it's a matter of applying the skill of problem solving to yourself. Your problem is the high tension. "How can I relax a little more?" And as I said, you also came up with the ideas yourself. It's really about setting a specific goal and then pursuing it. But maybe it will be a little easier if we plan it specifically together.

Difficulties that could arise with the problem-solving training method as well as suggested solutions are shown in Table 5.

Table 5. Potential difficulties and examples of therapeutic suggestions for the problem-solving intervention

Difficulties on the part of the caregivers	Behavior of the therapist
• Suggestions are ambivalent and none is exclusively positive or negative	• Suggest combinations of possible solutions • Have suggestions ranked • Motivate to make a preliminary decision about a current suboptimal solution
• Insufficient motivation to change	• Clarify values and long-term goals again
• General difficulty in making decisions and general uncertainty regarding goals	• Emphasize the provisional nature and the experimental character of the proposed solution • Point out that even attempts at coping can bring new information and thus optimize further attempts
• Unsuccessful problem-solving process	• Helpful self-reflection questions for therapists: • Was the description of the problem too imprecise? • Has a situation been selected that is not typical for the problem? • Were certain suggestions excluded hastily? • Was the wrong solution selected, i.e., a solution that did not lead to satisfactory coping with the stress or did not correspond to the actual desires? • Was the specific procedure not planned precisely enough that it was not really clear what to do? • Was the implementation of the steps too demanding? • Have potential difficulties been overlooked?

11.2.4 Reflecting the Implementation and Maintenance of Self-Care and Planned Pleasant Activities

Reflecting self-care activities

Therapist: You have started to take care of yourself.

Caregiver: Yes, yes, yes. Exactly.

Therapist: Yes, and do you slowly get the feeling that the shoe fits better, that it is no longer so unusual?

Caregiver: I think so [laughs].

Therapist: [laughs] It may not be a custom-made shoe, but it already feels better now.

Caregiver: It feels better [laughs]. Yes.

Caregivers should be asked continuously in the following sessions to reflect on their experiences in implementing more self-care and pleasant activities (see Questions 13). The therapist should reinforce every attempt at implementation and the caregivers should be given sufficient time to report on these experiences.

Questions 13. Reflecting on self-care and pleasant activities

- How have you been able to achieve incorporating pleasant activities the past week?
- How did you feel?
- What really did you good?
- How did you manage to do that?
- How did you overcome obstacles?
- Is there anything you'd like to do differently next time?

Difficulties in the implementation should be discussed in detail, and planned activities should be modified if it turns out that the activities cannot be realized under the given circumstances or that the caregivers do not feel comfortable enough with them. Above all, barriers such as *lack of time* should be discussed intensively. Caregivers often report that they have "forgotten" to do it or that there was no opportunity to carry out the pleasant activities in the stressful daily caregiving routine. At this point, the caregivers' personal values and needs should be discussed again and therapists should explore how important these really are to them and what consequences a nonrealization would have in the long term.

Therapists can encourage caregivers to stabilize the implementation of pleasant activities by having them consider and plan the implementation of the activities for the coming week at the end of each week. By informing family members or friends about the plans, the commitment to implement them can be strengthened further.

It has been helpful for activities that require an overnight stay away from home to make long-term plans with the caregivers, so that the person with dementia can be placed in a facility for short-term care or cared for by another family member. The exercise "My oasis day in each season," according to and translated to English for this manual (Kaluza, 2011, p. 95 ff.), can be used.

Therapeutic guidance: My oasis day in each season

Suppose you have gotten a taste for it and decide to do something good for yourself more often in the future. Then of course there is also the danger that this beautiful resolution will, so to speak, "go down the everyday stream" and vanish into oblivion. There is an effective antidote for this with the beautiful name, "Oasis day" or "four seasons project." The point is that you choose a specific place that you visit on four specific days of the year, either to withdraw from everything (that would then be an oasis day in the classic sense, where you are simply alone for a day or several days, for example in a hotel by the sea, or a nice walk in nature, or relaxing on your

---

Case Example 32. Guilty conscience

The following excerpt stems from therapy with a 61-year-old caregiving daughter.

Therapist: You said you have been caring for your mother for 11 years. That really is a very long time. It's very exhausting, it's very stressful emotionally. Suppose you've found the perfect nursing home and your mother's bags are packed. You bring your mother there, then suddenly she freezes. That can happen, you know.

Caregiver: Yes, that can happen. I've already thought about that.

Therapist: Yes, I ask because you said: "She comes first and she must feel well, and then I come second" – there is also a bit of risk involved with that, right?

Caregiver: Yes, that's right. And that is what others always say to me: "You have to think about yourself too," but I am not doing that at the moment. … But it's … Yes, I have always thought about others more and helped more than I have accepted help myself from others. And it has always been this way, even before I started taking care of my mother. It was always: "Do this … do that." I've always been there more for others, not for myself. And I can't just shed myself of that.

Therapist: That's probably something that developed relatively early on. How does it feel for you when you don't think of others first, but of yourself? What happens then?

Caregiver: Then I have a guilty conscience. Then I ruminate: "My goodness, if you had just …," and then it takes a long time until I say: "How come? I also have a right to certain things." Ultimately, I am entitled to my life too. Just like every other person has a right to all the comforts that every other person has a right to, I too have a right, regardless of whether my mother is sick or not. I know this, but I just can't shake it off.

Therapist: Yes, you really are quarreling with yourself.

Caregiver: Yes, yes, I am.

Therapist: You have a guilty conscience. You don't feel well with that. And yet you said, quite correctly, that you are also entitled to experience good years, that life goes on for you.

Caregiver: I think that often when I start ruminating and let the day pass. I think like this: "What did you have for yourself again today? Nothing, nothing at all." I would like to go on a trip for a few days again, go on a hike, just like I used to. Ultimately, they are modest desires, modest desires. Because I don't want to do a long-distance trip or anything.

Therapist: But just be away for a few days, relax, right?

Caregiver: Yes, exactly. But as I said, I know.

couch or recliner in the garden, or under a certain tree in the botanical garden), or to do something nice together with others. So now your task is to choose a place to go and also set the day, for example every first Wednesday in January, April, July, and October. And determine what you want to do that day. Your imagination is the limit.

The long-term goal of the therapeutic work should be for the caregivers to establish an attitude with which they are able to plan and undertake self-care behaviors and pleasant, value-oriented activities in the future and in their daily caregiving routine by themselves.

11.2.5 Dealing With a Guilty Conscience and Feelings of Guilt: Normalization and Acceptance

A major obstacle that family caregivers often state is a guilty conscience toward the person with dementia if they have done or would do something good for themselves. Many family caregivers live in an ambivalence between realizing their own needs and their own demands regarding caregiving. As soon as personal interests are pursued, caregivers appraise this as inconsideration toward the person with dementia and experience feelings of guilt. As a consequence, caregivers neglect the realization of their own needs (see Case Example 32).

Using disputation techniques, the long-term consequences of allowing their guilty conscience to prevent them from doing things for themselves should be illustrated. While doing so, it is important to point out that such feelings are normal and that many family caregivers experience them and that it is also a matter of accepting such unpleasant feelings (see Case Example 33).

In Case Example 33, Mrs. S. no longer participates in the Pilates class because she does not want to endure the feelings of guilt (or the thought "I am having fun here without my husband"). It becomes clear that tending to one's own needs (healthy, athletic lifestyle), as well as activities to realize one's own needs, is prevented by avoiding negative internal thoughts or feelings. Thus, there is a discrepancy between the caregiver's life goals and their implementation in everyday life. One reason for this in many cases is the tendency to avoid unpleasant internal experiences (negative feelings/thoughts/sensations). This has negative consequences: Avoidance leads to dissatisfaction and a negative mood in the long term and thus represents a potential trigger factor for overload or even mental illnesses such as depression or anxiety disorders. Therefore, behavior in the sense of avoidance is revealed by looking at planned activities that were not carried out and/or exploring neglected needs. At this point, it is very important to check objectively with the caregivers for each avoidance strategy (e.g., giving up Pilates class) whether it has helped them to feel better or what long-term consequences (costs) the avoidance behavior has or had. In most cases, strategies for avoiding negative feelings and thoughts are not effective in the long term.

During a walk with her friend, Mrs. S. experienced feelings of guilt again, that is, stopping the Pilates class (strategy for controlling thoughts of guilt) was unsuccessful in the long term. During the next self-care activities (going for a walk), the guilty thoughts reappear. If the caregivers find their previous strategies for avoiding certain emotions and thoughts helpful in the short term, the long-term costs of the behavior should be checked. *How will your life be if you keep avoiding your uncomfortable thoughts/feelings?* Based on the case example it becomes clear: If Mrs. S. continues evading her feelings of guilt, she will have to do without any activity connected to her value of "leading a healthy, athletic lifestyle." She will then probably only be able to cope with high blood pressure with the help of medication.

Case Example 33. Negative consequences of feelings of guilt

Mrs. S., 68 years old, has been caring for her husband suffering from dementia (75 years old) for 3 years. Before her husband became ill, the couple were very active athletically: both went jogging and sailing regularly. For Mrs. S. a "healthy athletic lifestyle" is an important need. But since Mr. S. fell ill, the couple's athletic activities have decreased a lot and by now Mrs. S. no longer exercises at all. She realizes that this is not good for her. Internally, she often feels very unbalanced, dissatisfied, and has gained weight. Now her family doctor has diagnosed her with high blood pressure and recommends that she starts exercising more again. Mrs. S.'s daughter has offered to look after her father one evening per week so that Mrs. S. can exercise. Mrs. S. has already found a Pilates class that is convenient in terms of time and location. However, after the first lesson, she reported to the therapist that she will no longer be attending the course. When asked why, she replied: "I would like to, but I had such a guilty conscience the whole time, I couldn't stand it."

In this context, therapists can convey to the caregivers that, overall, the attempt to avoid and control stressful thoughts and feelings is mostly unsuccessful. Box 18 contains an exercise that can be used to demonstrate to caregivers how difficult it is to control thoughts or emotions.

Box 18. Controlling thoughts is (quite) impossible

> The therapist asks the caregiver to concentrate for a minute on not thinking about a pink elephant (please really let the caregiver try it for a minute!). The experience is: The more one tries not to think about a pink elephant, the more difficult it becomes. The paradox can be explained by the fact that the thought, "I must not think about a pink elephant" already includes the pink elephant. This little exercise shows that controlling thoughts is (quite) impossible.

Afterwards, therapists can discuss with the caregivers acceptance of unpleasant feelings and thoughts. If caregivers cannot control feelings and thoughts (e.g., by quitting the Pilates class), and avoidance behavior prevents them from tending to their needs, then it is advisable for them to give up the avoidance behavior and to behave in line with their own needs. Importantly, caregivers should then accept associated negative feelings and thoughts. For Mrs. S. this means that she would go to the Pilates class *and* may experience feelings of guilt in doing so.

In order to avoid misunderstandings, it is important to discuss with the caregivers what exactly is meant by acceptance in this context. It is essential that acceptance is not used as a strategy to control unpleasant thoughts and feelings, but rather as a helpful way to live according to one's own needs. Acceptance is understood as an attitude of accepting positive and negative feelings and perceiving thoughts and sensations without wanting to change or avoid them. However, acceptance does not mean enduring or ignoring a changeable state.

Since caring for a person with dementia also entails an abundance of situations that are uncontrollable or only slightly controllable, due to the specific symptoms and progression of the syndrome, learning an accepting attitude beyond the subject of self-care is a necessary, but usually difficult, challenge for caregivers (see Chapter 12). In addition, it should be emphasized again and again that acting in line with one's own needs and "refueling" also serves the person with dementia. Most caregivers can even confirm this after their first experiences with pleasant activities. Caregivers often report that they were able to be more relaxed, balanced, and patient while in contact with the person with dementia (Case Example 34).

Case Example 34. Allowing self-care

The following excerpt stems from therapy with a 78-year-old caregiving wife.

Caregiver: Well, now I can reconcile that with my conscience. I wasn't able to do that in the past. I used to always think of it as pushing him away. And it took at least 6 months before I got over the fact that I'm not "pushing him away" when I put him in the day-care facility, but rather, that it's okay for both of us. Because he likes to go there. That's just it, he likes to go there.

Therapist: If you would put him in the day-care facility for a second day, what could you do on that day? How would that benefit you, and how would it maybe benefit him?

Caregiver: Yes, yes, for me it would be beneficial that I might actually be able to really *enjoy* the day. That I then say: "So, this is my day now." That I then go for a walk or visit a friend or something like that. I would do that on that day. Then I would *not* clean the house, but really only use the day for myself.

Therapist: How do you think you would feel in the evening after such a day?

Caregiver: Very good, yes, I would feel very good. Because I've shed myself of my guilty conscience. Since I no longer see it as pushing him away, I feel a little relieved on the days that he is no longer there. *That* has benefited me. I can go away: I close the door and nobody is there waiting. I'd have my peace. I would love to go to a café or even take longer hikes – I'd be able to do that then. And that would benefit me.

Therapist: And now imagine that you have this good feeling in the afternoon and your husband comes back from the day care – how could your good feeling have a positive effect on him?

Caregiver: That doesn't really have that effect on him. I've already noticed that. I pick him up, help him undress, and then I usually always take his bag right away and want to get it ready for the next time – then he often starts again and gets really aggressive again: "*No*, not the bag!" [Sigh] I have to explain to him again that I have to prepare his bag for the next time. He doesn't understand that at the moment. That's why he doesn't even notice that I'm a bit calmer at the beginning, or a bit more relaxed. Then that's gone right away. It's gone within a minute. Because it doesn't matter to him.

Therapist: And then we have the situation that he is more often aggressive in daily life, and my question is now aimed at where the difference could be? So, on the one hand, your husband is aggressive. You are quite tense one day because you haven't had time to do anything for yourself all day, but the other day you had time for yourself and are relatively relaxed – so what would be the difference in terms of your reaction to his aggressiveness in these two different situations?

Caregiver: Yes, then I don't react aggressively toward *myself*.

Therapist: Probably, right?

Caregiver: Yes, then I'm a bit too – I say: "Leave it!" [in a calm tone]. Then I try to keep myself under control. It is difficult, but I am trying.

Therapist: Great. So would that be a difference?

Caregiver: Yes, yes.

Therapist: So, you probably can't change his aggressive reaction, he won't notice whether you're relaxed or not, but what would probably be different is your reaction.

Caregiver: Yes, my reaction is different. That's it. Because I also notice when I have a day to myself and come home – even on the go, my God, I can enjoy things that I normally take care of on the run, and I notice this. I enjoy small things, for example visiting a friend, that's a given for everyone else, but for *us* it is not anymore.

Therapist: You then notice that you are doing a tremendous amount, Mrs. K., you are there for your husband around the clock, the nights are also difficult, you do not get much sleep, many things that you spontaneously feel like doing, you aren't able to do at all. So it is quite understandable that it's a very special experience for you when you can visit a friend.

Caregiver: The very first time my husband was in the day care, I went to the park. I love being out in nature. And then I sat down in a café by the pond, and thought: "Oh, now a nice cup of tea." I tried to enjoy it. Then I started to cry and thought: "My goodness, you're happy when you sit here and quietly have a cup of tea, when you're able to go for a short walk," which is for others, like we just said, is "a given." For us it's not anymore. Even if you want it to be. It simply does *not* work. That's why it's very, very nice for me to do something like this.

12 "From the Diagnosis Until Death" – Dealing With Change, Loss, and Grief

Examples. Caregivers mournful experiences of change and loss

> "And now his mental abilities are getting worse and worse. And when a person who is so familiar to you changes like that … it's very bitter … and I experience this every day. And every day I also have to make sure that I don't show him my sadness, because then he also gets very distraught."
>
> "And then I always think to myself: At some point, his impairment will end in death. For a year now, I've seen myself as a widow-to-be. This is very difficult for me, it makes me very sad."
>
> "We had so much planned for our life. And we still wanted to do so much and experience so many things … it's so sad."
>
> "We used to have such good conversations together. The saddest thing for me is the realization that I suddenly can no longer speak to him."
>
> "What especially hits me is the lack of thoughtfulness and affection that was very defining for our marriage."

Family caregivers live through continuous changes throughout the course of the syndrome and are faced with changing situations in which they have to reorient and reposition themselves. This requires a continuous adjustment process. Although most family caregivers notice changes long before the diagnosis is given, the time point of the dementia diagnosis can still trigger severe aggravation. Frequent reactions include shock, lack of perspective, fears for the future, symptoms of depression, discouragement, and sadness. These feelings can reoccur during phases in caregiving when changes or new situations arise. At the same time, some family members report a certain relief from the diagnosis since the problem behaviors can be attributed to and explained by a certain disorder.

The discrepancy between the generally unchanged physical appearance and the mental and personality-related changes in the person with dementia poses a perpetual and chronic burdensome situation for the family members. They must deal with the loss of the existing relationship and the mutual understanding of each other's roles and adapt to the associated changes.

The manner in which caregivers perceive and regulate their emotional reactions to the changes affects not only their coping with caregiving but also their subsequent adjustment process after the death of the person with dementia. Adequately dealing with the feelings that arise as a result of the changes can alleviate the perceived burden during caregiving and can also positively impact the later grieving process.

12.1 Goals of the Module

A multiconceptual treatment approach is required to support family caregivers in dealing with the changes in the personality of the person with dementia and the mutual relationship. The main goal is to improve the acceptance of new, unchangeable situations that arise as a result of the syndrome, and to accept the associated feelings. Family caregivers should be supported in recognizing the changes and losses associated with dementia and in learning to accept the new reality.

To achieve these goals, caregivers should be encouraged to deal with feelings (such as grief, guilt, and fears for the future). It is important to work on the perception, normalization, and acceptance of these feelings, and the new definition of one's role. Furthermore, by using cognitive techniques, burdensome thoughts related to the emerging feelings can be identified, and alternative thoughts can be developed. An additional goal is to (re-)activate resources that have not been used or that have been lost in order to facilitate caregivers in dealing with the burdensome feelings and experiences and, at the same time, to allow positive emotions. The family members should also be prepared for the time after the death of the person with dementia, and, if necessary, supported in their grieving process. Box 19 contains an overview of the interventions covered in this chapter.

Box 19. Overview of the interventions

> - Perceiving and expressing burdensome thoughts and feelings
> - Learning to accept burdensome thoughts and feelings
> - Identifying and processing dysfunctional thoughts in relation to emotional experiences
> - Working on redefining roles
> - Resource activation
> - Preparing for the death of the person with dementia
> - Support in the grieving process

12.2 Therapeutic Approach

An important task in therapeutic work with family caregivers is that they become aware of the changes caused by the illness and learn to understand and examine the associated thoughts and feelings (Example 17). Therefore, a nonjudgmental, empathetic therapeutic atmosphere is important, in which the family members can speak about their changed life situation as well as perceive and express their emotions.

Example 17. Allowing grief

> *Caregiver:* Yes, every now and then this sentence comes up: "It doesn't work anymore." Then she's aware of it.
>
> *Therapist:* And it goes without saying that your wife should be sad.
>
> *Caregiver:* Yes, of course. She takes a big look at me. I get teary-eyed, too. Then we both sit here and cry [laughs].
>
> *Therapist:* Yes, but that is also very important sometimes. Maybe it seems stupid and you have this feeling to fight against it.
>
> *Caregiver:* No, no, suppressing it leads to nothing.

12.2.1 Perceiving and Expressing Burdensome Thoughts and Feelings: Sadness, Guilt, and Anxiety

In order to prompt the caregivers to confront their burdensome thoughts and feelings, it can be helpful to ask them to describe the changes they experience in everyday life due to the disease, especially regarding their relationship with the person with the dementia and the person with dementia's personality (see Questions 14).

Questions 14. Exploring the changes

> - What has changed for you since your partner/your mother etc. fell ill?
> - How do you notice this change?
> - What feelings do you have in relation to the changes described?

Grief

Many caregivers find it difficult to perceive and express their grief due to changes such as the person with dementia's shift in personality or the loss of the mutual relationship. This is due to the fact that the person with dementia is still present but is constantly changing. Emerging feelings of grief are often perceived as inappropriate, or caregivers fear that they will encounter a lack of understanding from friends and family members if they openly express their feelings of sadness. However, suppressed sadness can also find another way out, for example, through physical tension or pain. It should be conveyed to the family caregivers that feelings of sadness due to the numerous and meaningful experiences of loss are normal and belong to the caregiving process. It is important that the therapist acknowledges and dignifies the suffering and pain endured due to the experience of loss (Example 18).

Example 18. Addressing grief

> *Caregiver:* If the weather was as nice as yesterday, in the past we would have said: "Come on, let's go to the park and take a nice walk." When you then realize: "Oh, that's not possible anymore" – then that's it. And it will never come back. Never.
>
> *Therapist:* How does that thought affect you, that it will never come back?

Caregiver: It makes me very sad. It makes me very sad. I've always said: "You can still teach small children something. You can't teach a person suffering from dementia anymore." I also know that the condition has *rapidly* declined in the last 3 months. Fast. And if it continues to decline so rapidly, then the situation will come that nothing is possible anymore.

Guilt

During the increasing depletion of the person with dementia's personal skills, but also after their death, feelings of guilt can arise in the family caregivers. On the one hand, this can exist in the sense of a *rational* or *real* guilt; for example, if there has been aggressive or negligent behavior toward the person with dementia, if apologies were not expressed while the person with dementia was still in a healthy state, or if one's own wrongdoings could not be resolved. In cases of real guilt, it is helpful for the caregivers to stand by it and acknowledge it. Family caregivers can be encouraged to express their guilt to the person with dementia, even if they can no longer accept or understand the apology. Feelings of guilt are, however, much more often *irrational* and can be related to thinking one should do more for the person with dementia or that one is partly to blame for the syndrome. Moreover, caregiving daughters often feel guilty about living out their own needs and utilizing various forms of support ("My mother has looked after me all her life, I can't put her in a day care").

The feeling of not being able to cope with the changes and their consequences can also be expressed in the form of desiring that the partner or parent suffering from dementia dies. The wish for his or her death as a form of liberation can, in turn, be linked to feelings of guilt (see Case Example 35).

> **Case Example 35. Feelings of guilt due to wishes for death**
>
> The following excerpt stems from therapy with a 59-year-old caregiving wife.
>
> *Therapist:* So what kind of specific thought comes to your mind?
>
> *Caregiver:* Oh [exhales] ... I'm taking him to the nursing home now.
>
> *Therapist:* I'm taking him to the nursing home now.
>
> *Caregiver:* Yes.
>
> *Therapist:* Okay. In the sense of, "I've reached my limit!"
>
> *Caregiver:* Now, yes, yes. ... So, yes. "I've reached my limit. I'll register him now for the nursing home." Or I've also thought: "If only he would die now."
>
> *Therapist:* Okay.
>
> *Caregiver:* That's *very* bad, isn't it?
>
> *Therapist:* Hmm.
>
> *Caregiver:* So, if it would just happen – but that would be best for all of us.
>
> *Therapist:* I'll repeat again: The thoughts are "I'm taking him to the nursing home now, I've reached my limit," or "It's been such a catastrophe, preferably, the easiest thing would be for him to die."
>
> *Caregiver:* Yes, yes. Then the decision would be made for me that I don't have to bring him away and he would no longer have to struggle.
>
> *Therapist:* And when you have these thoughts, how do you feel then? Which feelings do you have? What do you sense physically?
>
> *Caregiver:* Hmm ... well ... [exhales] ... I don't always feel better then. Sometimes worse, sometimes better, but mostly I think: "How could you think such a thing now?"

> *Therapist:* Is it perhaps that you are punishing yourself as a consequence? That you say to yourself: "How could you think such a thing now?"
>
> *Caregiver:* Yes.
>
> *Therapist:* If you look at it like this – "How could you think such a thing now?" – How are you then?
>
> *Caregiver:* Worse.
>
> *Therapist:* Hmm. Do you have feelings of guilt?
>
> *Caregiver:* Yes.

Caregiving partners often have so-called "survivor's guilt," which refers to the partner being ill and caregivers not allowing themselves to feel good about experiencing and doing nice things ("I simply can't allow myself to feel good right now while my husband is so sick, that's not how we both imagined our remaining years to be"). Case Example 39 in Section 12.2.4, deals with irrational guilt.

Fears for the Future and of the Person With Dementia's Death

By perceiving the progression of the syndrome, family caregivers are confronted not only with past and current perceived changes, but also with further losses and/or changes in the future that are linked to grief and worries. This can lead to fears for the future, which is above all associated with a feeling of helplessness.

Examples: Fears for the future

> "There comes this fear for the future, how it will all continue – because it has been happening rapidly lately. ... I'm really scared. I don't know if one day he won't recognize me anymore or something like that. How I am supposed to live here with him then?"

> "I always ask myself: Will I be able to do this if it continues?" you know? That's what I'm scared of. ... And there are so many fears. After all, there is not just fear about my husband's state of health. There is the fear, the fear for the future, "What shall we do, the two of us, when we are alone?" There are so many ... fears that connect to one another and to make matters worse, he has recently started to become really aggressive, which is something that many people have told me could happen. But I didn't really expect that to happen so quickly because he has actually never done that until now. Let's hope I can get through this. That I – that I don't react differently somehow. So, I'm scared of that too. You don't even know yourself."

> "I notice my fear of loneliness more and more, and already right now since I can no longer talk to my husband at all. I'm actually not used to living alone, and the thought of being all alone once my husband has died really bothers me. Assuming my husband will be dead in 4 years, I think to myself: "How will you be doing?" and yes ... sometimes, lately I've been worrying about that. And I also imagine not being able to get by on my own and then I might make decisions that aren't good for me, for example, rushing into a new relationship too quickly."

Difficult future decisions, especially regarding nursing-home placement of the partner or parent suffering from dementia, also represent a great burden. At the same time, adjusting to the time after death is also frightening – caregiving spouses especially fear not being able to cope well with life alone. Strong anxiety can have a massive impact on the daily caregiving routine, can be paralyzing, and can limit the possibilities to react and act appropriately in current situations. Family caregivers often avoid confronting the future, because they find it to be a topic that is too burdensome. Typically, this can be observed by caregiving children in the early stage of the parent's syndrome, and in caregiving partners in the middle stage of the partner's illness (Meuser & Marwit, 2001). However, confrontation with the future is important, and should be encouraged by the therapist.

Planning the future strengthens the family caregivers' experience of control and enables them to acquire problem-solving skills and organize informal as well as professional support. The therapist's task should be to reinforce the caregivers' trust in their own strengths, as well as to encourage coping strategies and realistic expectations for the future (see further instructions and case examples in Chapter 14).

12.2.2 Confronting and Coping With Feelings of Grief, Guilt, and Anxiety

Most caregivers find it easy to talk about the changes in everyday life but have difficulties confronting their emotions associated with those changes. Uncomfortable feelings are mostly avoided or suppressed. Caregivers should be told that experiencing various burdensome feelings such as grief, anxiety, and guilt in the face of the constant changes is a normal and important process; suppressing or avoiding these feelings does not lead to a reduction of the emotional state but rather reinforces them. Moreover, attempts to cope with unpleasant feelings can also involve problems and have a negative effect on mood, for example, when caregivers constantly preoccupy themselves with the unpleasant feelings (e.g., through burdensome brooding). Psychoeducation 13 shows how feelings can occur.

Psychoeducation 13. Our array of feelings

> Feelings are an important part of our lives. In particular, unpleasant feelings have a signal function. It is therefore important to give attention to our feelings. Sometimes we have become accustomed to treating unpleasant feelings as something disturbing and pushing them aside as much as possible, avoiding them, or denying them. Perhaps we find it difficult to show our feelings openly in the presence of others because we fear that they will overwhelm our counterparts or because we have had unpleasant experiences in the course of our lives when we openly admit sadness, anger, or fear in front of others. That is how we have learned to hold back these feelings. This may have made it easier for us to cope with our environment. The disadvantage, however, is that we later found it difficult to perceive and sense our feelings. Most unpleasant feelings, however, play an extremely important role in our lives. If we are not aware of our own feelings, we also have no indication of what is good for us and what is not. This is why it is important that we take the time to observe uncomfortable feelings, explore them, and recognize their signals. We can most likely change unpleasant feelings if we first open ourselves to our emotional experiences and accept them.

In the therapy sessions, avoidance of emotions is shown in different behaviors: Family caregivers divert from emotional topics by starting a successive flow of speech or leading an intellectualized confrontation. Moreover, in face-to-face sessions, caregivers often avoid eye contact and have a tense posture.

In these cases, it is necessary to address the avoidance behavior directly: "Do you find it difficult to talk about your experience?" "I noticed that you went astray from my actual question. Could that be because it is not easy for you to talk about your feelings and sensations?" Case Example 36 addresses avoidance behavior.

For a better visualization, the therapist can ask the family caregivers to imagine pushing an air-filled balloon under water. This image should make clear that avoiding or suppressing unpleasant feelings leads to them reappearing. For a neurophysiological explanation of this process of persistent activation of problematic emotions, see Lammers (2011, p. 103).

For family caregivers who have difficulties accessing their own feelings, it can be helpful to discuss with them which feelings can be differentiated as well as the functions of our feelings. In addition, Worksheet 12-1: List of Our Feelings (according to Lammers, 2011, p. 337) can be used.

Family caregivers should learn to experience their emotions consciously and to avoid them no longer. In this context, the family caregivers will be informed that accepting the changes in their life situation and the associated feelings has a favorable effect on their psychological and physical well-being.

Family caregivers are therefore instructed to sense and verbalize their emotions. The following questions can be helpful in this process:
- "What exactly do you feel when you are talking about it?"
- "What do you feel when you think about …/imagine …?"
- "How does your body feel when you talk about …?"

The avoidance behavior can be abolished if the therapist continuously addresses and names the family caregivers' emotions and directs the caregivers to their emotional senses. However, this should always be done in a dosed manner so that the caregivers can experience talking about feelings without being overwhelmed by them.

12.2.3 Accepting Thoughts and Feelings

The awareness of changes caused by the syndrome and the inevitability of the impending death alternate with denial of the fact that the person with dementia continues to change and the disease is incurable.

> **Case Example 36. Emotional avoidance**
>
> The following excerpt stems from therapy with an 82-year-old caregiving husband.
>
> *Caregiver:* There's really no situation where I just sit there and let myself think. But I don't see that as a problem either.
>
> *Therapist:* Sometimes, it can be helpful to devote yourself to your thoughts. You're in a situation right now where there are a lot of changes.
>
> *Caregiver:* Yes, yes, that's true.
>
> *Therapist:* And perhaps your feelings are also changing?
>
> *Caregiver:* Yes, they are.
>
> *Therapist:* How would you describe these feelings?
>
> *Caregiver:* Above all, they are uncomfortable. I can't really describe it. Basically, everything has changed for me. There are so many feelings, uncomfortable ones.
>
> *Therapist:* Do you sometimes give space to these unpleasant feelings? Are there moments when you give your attention to these feelings, or is it more so that you try to repress them, to suppress them?
>
> *Caregiver:* Actually, I try to suppress them, I have … that's changed a bit. Well, that's what I've done before. One always has some worries, and then I just let myself go, for about an hour, and then afterwards I notice the release of tension. There's a physical relaxation effect, in a certain way. But that was in the past, now I find it kind of inappropriate. I mean … my wife, she is still there … I can't …
>
> *Therapist:* What do you mean exactly?
>
> *Caregiver:* I don't want to … and I also notice that this might make me have thoughts or feelings that aren't desirable at all.
>
> *Therapist:* Hmm, which feelings do you mean?
>
> *Caregiver:* That it's no longer the way it was. That everything is changing, and that thoughts and feelings arise that I actually forbid myself to have since my wife is still here.
>
> *Therapist:* Which feelings and thoughts do you forbid yourself to have?
>
> *Caregiver:* Well, I don't know if it's appropriate, but it's grief, I've actually been saying goodbye for a long time, and I'm sometimes ashamed of it, because then I think to myself, she's still here.

The difficulties caregivers have in accepting existing changes or negative feelings are illustrated by their frequent searching for new solutions and compensatory possibilities for the developing deficits of the person with dementia, for example, by following current studies on the cure of dementia, asking physicians for new medication prescriptions, doing cognitive or motor exercises with the person with dementia on a daily basis, or attributing changes in the person with dementia's personality to external events such as the weather (see Case Example 6, "Lack of acceptance of the illness," in Chapter 5). By adopting a more accepting attitude, family caregivers can obtain new energy and thus make changes in their lives that facilitate an adequate adjustment process. In addition, this can prevent the person with dementia from being overstrained by family caregivers (e.g., inadequate cognitive or motor training, setting tasks that can no longer be mastered, excessive communication; see also Case Example 15, "Guided discovery to encourage understanding the person with dementia," in Chapter 9). The family caregivers should be supported in allowing and accepting these emotions (see Example 19).

Example 19. Accepting uncomfortable sensations

> The following excerpt stems from therapy with a 57-year-old caregiving wife.
>
> *Therapist:* When you sit alone on the couch in the evening, exhausted from the day, and you have already put your husband to bed, what do you think at that moment?

Caregiver: Then I think, "I can't take all of this anymore. I want my old life back."

Therapist: And do these thoughts help you at this moment?

Caregiver: Mm-hmm, probably not, but then I just want all of it to come to an end, for everything to be like it used to be. When I have these thoughts, I feel a lot of pressure in my chest.

Therapist: Could it be that you are fighting a bit against the feeling that is there at that moment? That you cannot accept that a lot has changed and that there are many negative aspects associated with it?

Caregiver: Yes, but one can't accept that. Then I'd have the feeling that I'm falling into an even deeper hole.

Therapist: That is often the fallacy that we assume. Actually, it's exactly the other way around. Fighting against it usually increases the feeling. If we manage to let in our negative feelings and accept that they are there, our tension will be reduced.

Caregiver: I would have to try that sometime.

Therapist: Yes, maybe you can say to yourself, "There is this feeling now that's part of me right now. I try to accept it. It belongs to my current state, and I allow it."

In order to be able to accept and process the changes involved with the disease, the acceptance of painful feelings is, as already described, an important step. However, this is usually a lengthy process.

In the therapy dialogue in Case Example 37, a distinction between different feelings is worked out with the help of a preceding problem analysis (not fully printed, the dialogue begins at the end of the problem analysis). On this basis, it is easier for the family caregiver to gain understanding and clarity about their feelings and to accept them.

In our experience, additional small mindfulness exercises such as those in the manual by Reddemann (2020) have proven to be helpful in allowing and perceiving painful emotions (see Box 20).

The visualization in Box 20 promotes a more conscious awareness of emotions and physical sensations in the family caregivers. This also enables better access to one's own needs and thus creates an important prerequisite for the implementation of desired changes.

Box 20. Short mindfulness exercise (according to Reddemann, 2020)

> I ask you now to find a posture that's comfortable for you. ... First, feel that your body is in contact with the floor. It's all about perceiving that your body has contact and where it has contact. It's not about right or wrong but about consciously perceiving. ... And next, I ask you to perceive that your body is breathing and that it is making certain movements in the process. Notice these movements. Notice that the chest rises and falls gently. ... And that the abdominal wall rises and falls. ... And if you pay attention very closely, you will feel the nostrils making very small movements. Perceive these movements of the body while breathing for a few moments. ... End the exercise by becoming aware again that your body is in contact with the chair and perceive your physical boundaries mindfully. Then return your attention to the room and consciously perceive this.

12.2.4 Identifying and Processing Dysfunctional Thoughts in Relation to Emotional Experiences

Perceiving, expressing, and accepting feelings can be made more difficult by dysfunctional thought patterns.

Examples: Dysfunctional thoughts related to emotional experience

> - "My family member suffering from dementia is still there, I am not allowed to show any mourning yet."
> - "If I allow my sadness, I fear that I will become depressed."
> - "If I allow all of that, I will fall into a deep hole."
> - "Dealing with fears for the future just makes me even more afraid."
> - "If I think about all of the things I can no longer do because of caregiving, it will only get worse."
> - "I mustn't be angry that he leaves me on my own with everything here. He doesn't deserve that."
> - "If I accept all of these changes and negative feelings, then I'll have the feeling that I've given up, that I just won't be able to function anymore."

By using the methods of cognitive restructuring (see Case Example 38), when indicated in connection with psychoeducation, family caregivers can learn to recognize these paralyzing and discouraging thoughts and to develop al-

Case Example 37. Distinguishing and accepting feelings

The following excerpt stems from therapy with a 77-year-old caregiving wife.

Therapist: What are your first thoughts on the problem analysis we just did? Can you already draw something from it?

Caregiver: No, I still don't know exactly how to deal with him.

Therapist: By analyzing the problematic situation, we found out that telling him that he is demented is not at all a burden for you, but when he ignores you, you then feel alone, and get sad and angry.

Caregiver: Yes, yes.

Therapist: Separating that would be the first important point for me. The way I see the current situation, the bad feelings come up not because you did something wrong, but because you are hurt at that moment.

Caregiver: Mm-hmm ... yes. Correct.

Therapist: I have the feeling that your feelings of sadness and anger are not a sign that you did something wrong, but a reaction to experiencing loss in the situation. How you feel is not evidence that you are doing something wrong in the situation. Can you find any sense in what I am saying?

Caregiver: Yes, at that moment, it was all mixed up. I wasn't sure if it was okay that I was so open about the word "demented."

Therapist: Yes. That is also very understandable. At that moment, thoughts flash through your head in a matter of seconds, and the feelings are mixed? But if we make sense of that now, it turned out that it is not the dissatisfaction with your reaction that is at the center of attention, but rather the sadness about your husband ignoring you.

Caregiver: Yes. I'm thinking about it right now. That was last night. Until then, I was also, I was also really calm. I was able to talk to him about it, but from the moment he ignored me, I know this situation from before. Then you have to deal with it.

Therapist: Before, you had dealt with the situation very calmly. You explained it to him objectively, and when he then ignored you, these feelings came. And this is something that you're familiar with.

Caregiver: Yes. He doesn't ask me either. Like how I'm doing, or "Why are you crying?" or something like that. Not at all.

Therapist: Yes. That means that it is very important that your feelings do not tell you that you did something wrong at the moment. But that you felt alone in the moment?

Caregiver: Mm-hmm. Yes.

Therapist: That means, in this situation, the key topic is loneliness?

Caregiver: Yes. Yes.

Therapist: Yes. Mm-hmm. And that is something that I hear in your voice, that it's a difficult topic.

Caregiver: Yes ...

Therapist: Mm-hmm. Does it help you when we look at it so closely?

Caregiver: I think that it helps me. And, you know, I would like to be able to deal with it differently. These situations will happen again and again, I already know that, you know.

Therapist: Exactly. Yes. Although I think it's okay for the moment when you go out and are sad and then cry too.

Caregiver: Mm-hmm.

Therapist: You have not behaved wrongly toward your husband by doing that.

Caregiver: No. It's just, when I am sad about it, I would actually like for him to ask me, "What is it? Don't we want to talk about it?" that he tries to comfort me or at least tells me: "It's okay now, I didn't mean it like that" or something. And he doesn't even notice that I am feeling bad at the moment.

Therapist: That is to say, it's a new situation. That when you are sad, that a consoling or comforting gesture is missing.

Caregiver: Exactly.

Therapist: To know, that he actually is no longer able to do it, and on the other hand, to have the need and to not be able to accept it.

Caregiver: Yes.

Therapist: If you look at it so closely. Because in principle, this is a fundamental conflict that we have already discussed and that has come up again.

Caregiver: Yes, exactly. Yes, that really old things have come up again.

Therapist: Yes, this feeling of loss and loneliness.

Caregiver: Yes. Yes.

Therapist: Yes. But I find that you really took an important step today, even though it is difficult for you. You really did great today. To understand for the first time what exactly happens in the situation, to understand for the first time why the feelings are so strong in the situation.

Caregiver: Mm-hmm. Mm-hmm.

Therapist: That is the first step in order to get a little distance from the feeling.

Caregiver: Yes.

Therapist: Yes, and maybe in the next situation to say: "Okay, I know this feeling."

Caregiver: That I really, that I can deal with it differently, with him ignoring me. That's just the way it is, and I've been through this before, I'm familiar with this. It's nothing new for me.

Therapist: Yes. A helpful thought for example would be: "Okay, now the old feeling is coming up again, I've been here before, and for the moment it's just there, but I already know it. I don't have to be overwhelmed by it."

Caregiver: Yes, to not feel so hurt anymore, you know. Oomph, you get pounded on the head. So now I go, I'm familiar with such a feeling, I've been here before and then it's okay.

Therapist: Yes. I think that's a good, good train of thought. Because we probably won't be able to get rid of the feeling.

Caregiver: It is there. You can't suppress feelings.

Therapist: Unfortunately, there is no magic wand for that.

Caregiver: Nope, that doesn't exist.

Therapist: Mm-hmm. And I also think it's important that your bad feelings are not proof that you have done something wrong and that you always have to look closely at it.

Caregiver: Yes.

Therapist: Exactly. Do you have any more questions or thoughts about this, is there still something on your mind?

Caregiver: I only notice that I have become much calmer. I guess because of what we talked about.

Case Example 38. Cognitive restructuring on the subject of grief

The following excerpt stems from therapy with a 70-year-old caregiving wife.

Caregiver: Yes, you have to watch yourself too. It's actually really difficult that I'm so alone now, sometimes I fall into such a deep hole, but in the end I always get out of it. It works out somehow.

Therapist: I have the feeling a bit that you are afraid of allowing yourself to mourn. That it somehow shouldn't be. That you have to distract and occupy yourself immediately and put the grief aside. What do you fear would happen to you if the grief occurred?

Caregiver: Yes, I'm afraid then that – I've heard from others – that I will become depressed and will no longer be able to take care of my husband. I don't want that. I want my husband to be at home and that I maybe hire someone. These are all things that I have to try to sort out, and also that maybe two people come, so that I might be able to go away for a few days or so. Get away completely.

Therapist: That would be really good. Yes. How was that before – I mean, every journey through life has phases of sadness and loss of some kind – how did you deal with sadness or grief in the past? Are you familiar with these feelings?

Caregiver: Yes. My father, he also died very badly. He fought hard for 6 weeks. He had a heart attack and then pneumonia. And that's when I stopped working and, in the end, I actually stayed with him until his death.

Therapist: That was also very strenuous for you.

Caregiver: Yes, I also had enormous problems afterward. I almost couldn't laugh. It was weird. I wasn't at all … it was a long process, this sadness that I had, especially with my father.

Therapist: Does your fear of becoming depressed come from that?

Caregiver: Yes, I'm a little afraid. That I will get depressed.

Therapist: Does that come from the experience, "I couldn't laugh at all for a long time?"

Caregiver: I have an aunt who was also depressed. She had her mother at home, and she could actually no longer care for her at home because she became depressed and then gave her to the nursing home. And then I saw it so closely and … I don't want this to happen to me.

Therapist: Hmm.

Caregiver: That is my fear.

Therapist: Depression has a lot to do with a feeling of emptiness. If people can express emotions, it is somehow something vital. So, there is something vital about being able to express sadness. So, I don't think that this fear of becoming depressed when you experience sadness is conclusive. … Sadness is more of a healthy sign. Well, it would be strange if you had to say goodbye to certain things that you have in common with your husband and feel nothing.

Caregiver: That it wouldn't touch me …

Therapist: Exactly. But it's okay to be sad; it's a perfectly normal reaction. In this way, you are also processing the situation a little.

Caregiver: Maybe I see it a different way. That you always have this fear: "No, you mustn't do that now … you have to see …" and then I push certain things aside.

Therapist: That sounds like a lot more pressure to me. When I am sad and I say to myself: "I'm not supposed to be sad at all. I have to function here now, and I have to distract myself, and I have to do this and that." Sounds like additional pressure to me.

Caregiver: Yes, yes.

Therapist: Additional energy that you need there. That's why I think it's okay if you have an evening where you're sad, crying, and then say to yourself: "Okay, today I can grant myself a couple hours of sadness." I think that's really okay.

Caregiver: Hmm … yes, maybe I have to deal with it differently in the future. Tell myself that I won't get depressed from it.

Therapist: Just try what is good for you, but I don't think that you have to be terrified of becoming depressed when you feel sad. This is a perfectly normal and healthy reaction. This is important. How difficult is it for you to talk about it now, because earlier it really touched you, as far as I could tell, on the phone …

Caregiver: [laughs] Yes, now I'm somehow better again when you tell me that one can allow it and that one does not need to be this afraid … that makes me feel better.

Therapist: This train of thought helps you more than the thought that you could become depressed?

Caregiver: Yes, absolutely, it makes me feel better.

At the end of the session:

Therapist: How did you find our talk today? Did you take a little something for yourself?

Caregiver: Certainly. Yes, definitely. What you've told me that one can allow this grief and that one won't get depressed right away. So, I thought about the fact that maybe one should allow it more. Doesn't mean that one has to cry for hours or so, but that you have to just say to yourself: "It's not bad, it's just the way it is and it can be."

Case Example 39. Irrational feelings of guilt

The following excerpt stems from therapy with a 60-year-old caregiving wife.

Caregiver: Thoughts often appear when I think about my husband's life. He practically worked all his life and … actually he deserves something else. That his life ends with such an illness is, of course, depressing when you think about it: The one person you are connected to and then who gets into this situation … and I myself feel relatively well. Sometimes I have the feeling that … that I'm practically sucking the life out of him, if you will. It's such a strange feeling, I don't even really want to let it get to me.

Therapist: Is it a type of feeling of guilt of being the stronger one, a survivor's guilt?

Caregiver: Yes. I've sometimes asked myself if I had any part in it, if I was to blame for his dementia, and I've tried to read about whether there are factors that can influence the development of such an impairment, you know?

Therapist: Yes, and what did you come across?

Caregiver: Well, actually I haven't found anything in that direction. Actually, that it's an illness that occurs and that isn't due to previous psychological stress. I mean, we've been together for 30 years and of course my husband has a different nature than I do. I'm naturally calmer.

Therapist: Yes.

Caregiver: And sometimes I had the impression that perhaps he needs someone who's a little more animated than I am, and that perhaps he missed that. Now sometimes, the thought comes to mind that his impairment is due to him having to do without a lot of things because of me. He never said this, but I thought that maybe he had thoughts like that after all, maybe it had an effect. But then I heard a lecture from a physician …

Therapist: Yes, you said that you were there.

Caregiver: And then I specifically asked about it, and he also said that there are no external factors that make it happen.

Therapist: Do you believe that if you had taken more action or if your husband had had another wife that this disease would not have happened?

Caregiver: That's the exact question that I asked myself. And of course you can't tell now, it's just the way it is. And we can't do an experiment now where it would be different.

Therapist: But the question is, what does a thought like that do to you? Which feeling does this thought provoke?

Caregiver: It gnaws at me ... made me think that maybe I did something wrong.

Therapist: Mm-hmm, I understand. Does that help you right now?

Caregiver: Of course, it doesn't help me, no, not at all. That's it, that's the problem. These are thoughts that have a negative effect and that I would rather not have.

Therapist: Hmm, exactly. This thought leads to you feeling guilty.

Caregiver: This statement that there are no external factors calmed me down a bit, but ...

Therapist: Yes. How high would you rate the probability that the disease would not have broken out under different living conditions?

Caregiver: Hmm, very low, very.

Therapist: What would indicate that your husband was unhappy with you in your marriage?

Caregiver: Yes, actually there aren't that many things [laughs]. I think that by and large it was okay, but the thought came up, I have to say.

Therapist: Hmm. Would your husband have had the opportunity to split up if he had been unhappy?

Caregiver: Yes, of course ...

Therapist: Was that ever an issue?

Caregiver: No, of course there were arguments, but it was never seriously considered that we wanted to break up.

Therapist: Does this thought that your husband never considered the subject of separation change anything about your feeling that he was unhappy and could have become ill with dementia as a result?

Caregiver: Yes, it makes me feel a little relieved.

ternative, potentially more helpful thoughts (for corresponding intervention techniques of Socratic dialogue and the ABC model, see also Chapter 8).

In all cases of irrational guilt (see Case Example 39), the technique of cognitive restructuring is suitable to explore the thoughts on which the feelings of guilt are based and to check their degree of reality.

12.2.5 Working on Redefining Roles

Due to the dementia of the partner or one of the parents, the balance that has developed over the course of a long-standing marital or parental relationship is disturbed. The taking on of new roles by the healthy family member not only overloads the caregiver, but the person with dementia also increasingly loses their autonomy. Because the person with dementia's appearance barely changes over the course of the syndrome, the caregiver is, therefore, often reminded of how the relationship used to be. Therefore, redefining the relationship and dealing with the changes that have been made and are to be expected are essential goals in therapy with family caregivers. This redefinition is intended to protect caregivers against unrealistic expectations toward the person with dementia, which in turn can heavily burden and impair the relationship. Changes in the relationship between the caregiver and the person with dementia should be explored (see Questions 15) and, if necessary, new role definitions should be found.

Questions 15. Redefining roles

- How do you feel about your marital relationship right now? Do you have the impression that the roles have changed?
- How do you feel as a daughter right now? Can you still be a daughter or do you have the feeling that something has changed in your role?
- How else could one describe your current relationship? Also, could you find a term for it other than mother–daughter relationship?

The goal of therapy is first to explore what changes the new role will involve, as well as possible advantages and disadvantages that could result. It is also important that the skills and support that the new role requires are discussed and developed. The family caregivers should gain certainty and self-confidence in dealing with the changed roles and obtain assurance that they will be able to cope (see Case Examples 40 and 41).

Case Example 40. Redefining roles

The following excerpt stems from therapy with a 47-year-old caregiving daughter.

Therapist: How would you define your role at the moment? Do you feel like you are living in a mother–child relationship?

Caregiver: No, not anymore. Now it's more like the other way around, so that I take on the role of mother and my mother ... she's just like a child sometimes. Well, the roles are different now.

Therapist: And what does that mean for living together when the roles are different now?

Caregiver: That I can't expect certain things anymore and that I also have responsibility now. That I can no longer rely on her advice. And I also have to make decisions for her.

Therapist: And how are you doing with that?

Caregiver: Yes, it's a big change. It's not always easy for me either. For example, she doesn't want to go to day care. She protests every time and then we argue. I can't leave her at home alone. There's the one day that I do the bookkeeping in my husband's company. But every time she says that she can stay home alone. You know, and then I just make the decision for her that she has to go there. That doesn't feel good either. I always have a guilty conscience. She is my mother, you know, she also has her own will. And then I think to myself ... it's just not right for you to just decide over her head. Are you even allowed to do that?

Therapist: Mm-hmm ... I understand. If you look at it in the context of what you described earlier ... that you now have the role of the mother. How did you do that with your children in the past? Where there days where your children didn't want to go to Kindergarten?

Caregiver: [laughs] Yes, there were.

Therapist: And what did you do then?

Caregiver: I gently coaxed them into going. Told them they had to go. They had to go, I had to work.

Therapist: In other words, you just made the decision.

Caregiver: Yes.

Therapist: And did you have a guilty conscience about it?

Caregiver: Not really. They were too young to make good decisions themselves.

Therapist: And how is it now with your mother? Would you say she can still make good decisions?

Caregiver: No, she can't anymore. I wouldn't have any peace at all if she were home alone.

Therapist: As if you had left your children at home alone in the past.

Caregiver: Exactly ... now I see what you're getting at. I have to get used to this role first, but of course, that's part of it, that I make decisions for her because she is no longer good at it. And that I don't really have to have a guilty conscience.

Therapist: Yes, exactly, because the roles are different now.

> **Case Example 41. Redefining roles**
>
> The following excerpt stems from therapy with a 71-year-old caregiving wife.
>
> *Caregiver:* Sometimes I treat him like a child and then I always feel really bad. I think: "You can't be in charge of him like that."
>
> *Therapist:* Yes, of course, you don't want that in a marriage.
>
> *Caregiver:* Yes, I don't want that, but somehow there is no other way sometimes.
>
> *Therapist:* The relationship has probably changed a lot? It's not like it used to be?
>
> *Caregiver:* Yes [cries].
>
> *Therapist:* That's painful.
>
> *Caregiver:* Yes.
>
> *Therapist:* Do you still feel equally as husband and wife?
>
> *Caregiver:* That's a good question [contemplates]. Do you know what I think sometimes? It would probably be better if I could get to the point that I'm the nurse and he's the patient.
>
> *Therapist:* Would looking at it that way make the situation easier for you?
>
> *Caregiver:* Yes, somehow. I think it describes how I feel.
>
> *Therapist:* What would change if you take on this mindset?
>
> *Caregiver:* Then it is somehow okay that I am now responsible for everything and can also be in charge. Then I expect less from him. Then the roles are somehow more clearly assigned.
>
> *Therapist:* Yes, I think that's a good thought.

12.2.6 Resource Activation

In the above-mentioned intervention strategies, emotion-focused interventions to facilitate the process of allowing negative feelings were emphasized. Adequately dealing with emotions can be seen as an important resource. Because there are many reasons for the family caregiver's negative or painful feelings, the goal is to develop new possibilities for dealing with these feelings. This takes time and works only if the painful feelings are accepted. In addition, positive feelings should also be (re-)activated in caregivers, as these facilitate coping with the constant changes and losses.

Thus, in the therapy sessions, family caregivers should be given the opportunity to relive their positive characteristics and abilities and to use these in order to perceive and satisfy their own needs. It is important to promote self-efficacy with regard to coping with existing problem areas. In this context, it can be helpful to ask how difficult life situations were dealt with in the past and/or how the family caregivers managed to cope well despite the many difficulties (see Questions 16).

Questions 16. Resource activation

- How have you dealt with difficult changes in your life so far?
- How was it in the past – how did you deal with grief, anxiety, or feelings of guilt? Are you familiar with this from other situations?
- What could you say to yourself to cope with the situation better? Do you have any ideas?
- Which thoughts or feelings give you strength/help you in dealing with your situation better?
- How have you managed to cope so well despite the difficult situation?
- What is currently going so well in your life that you don't want to change it?

It can always be helpful to see positive aspects in the current situation or to consciously address positive things. Thus, family caregivers can be asked to do things they find comfortable or encouraged to consciously avert themselves from worries and devote a few moments to positive experiences.

It also proves to be important to remember positive moments from the past with the person with dementia and to consider which joyful or satisfying moments occur in the current phase in life (see Questions 17). Despite the many changes and the mental and physical decline of the person with dementia, most family caregivers are able to see and remember current moments of happiness.

Questions 17. Recalling moments of joy

- Which happy moments together can you remember?
- Moments of happiness can exist even in the saddest phases in life. Are there still moments today where you feel joy with them or that make you feel satisfied?

To improve one's own resources, support from the family or professionals can also be activated in order to provide more relief (see Chapter 13). Such relief creates space to deal with one's own feelings and needs in order to be able to process the changing life situation better and reduce stress. In addition, family caregivers should be encouraged to confide in other people (friends, family members) and to share their experiences regarding the changes in order to counteract feelings of isolation or hiding feelings of sadness. Chapter 11 contains further strategies for resource activation.

12.3 The Time After the Death of the Person With Dementia

Although it is not necessary in most cases to provide therapeutic support for the aftermath of a human loss and the associated grief reactions, since most people manage to adapt to the loss, supportive therapeutic talks with family caregivers can still be helpful. For many family caregivers, at the end of caregiving, a task that has been important for them and that has stabilized their self-esteem is eliminated. Thus, it can be helpful to accompany family caregivers during this adjustment process and in creating new life goals. The support described above for dealing with the mourning process can also be helpful for coping with the loss. Psychoeducational interventions, such as an introduction to the demands of grief, can also be helpful. Further literature on this topic can be found for example by Worden (2018). There is currently much controversy among scientists about the topic of therapeutic support for bereavement. Thus far, no psychotherapeutic guidelines have been formulated, meaning that therapists should take the greatest care while addressing bereavement with the family caregivers. Therapeutic talks

> **Case Example 42. Helpful rituals for dealing with the experience of loss**
>
> The following excerpt stems from therapy with a 63-year-old caregiving daughter.
>
> *Caregiver:* Well, by and large, the trip was of course great, but then I always thought about my mother. I, this might sound absurd, but I took one of her necklaces with me and wore it and somehow that gave me a bit of a bond.
>
> *Therapist:* I don't find that absurd at all, rather it's a … good strategy that you have already used for yourself. Well, that you use a symbol that reminds you of your mother to establish a connection to her. I believe that is something very positive that you have done for yourself.
>
> *Caregiver:* I had never considered telling anyone else about it. I thought they would think: "She's crazy!"
>
> *Therapist:* Hmm. No, well, in therapy, we work with symbols very often. That one uses such small objects that one connects with something, to process something, or to remember something, and you intuitively did that very well for yourself. To create an inner closeness, to deal with the sadness. That's a really great thing you've done, to use a symbol like the necklace your mother used to wear herself.
>
> *Caregiver:* And I lit a candle in M.
>
> *Therapist:* As a ritual for you, to think about her.
>
> *Caregiver:* Yes.
>
> *Therapist:* That is something really wonderful, because you gave yourself space, so to speak. The time that you take to think exclusively about her. This is a very good strategy that you have already used intuitively. If something accompanies you all day, be it worries, sadness, or something nice, for instance, that you want to think of something, then it is good to say: "Okay, I'll make time for it when it's time to do it. I'll give myself a half hour to think about it very intensely, to worry or be sad about it." To create such a time window. When you notice that you are feeling overwhelmed, then you can say: "I have my half hour, that's when I'll take time for it."

should by no means be forced, but instead it should be considered together with the family caregivers whether a therapeutic accompaniment for bereavement is desired and what it might look like.

Case Example 42 describes how a caregiving daughter deals with her mother's death. The therapist reinforces the daughter's successful coping strategies.

12.3.1 Consequences of Anticipatory Grief

As a consequence of the adjustment process described so far and the constant confrontation with feelings of loss and grief, caregiving family members already go through a process that can be classified as equivalent to the adjustment process after the death of a person (anticipatory grief). It is not uncommon for this adjustment process to lead to the absence of the expected grief reaction after the death of the person with dementia. This is the case when the phases of grief have already been experienced, and emotional detachment from the deceased has already occurred. Due to the person with dementia's cognitive impairments, family caregivers do not generally experience shared grief with the person with dementia, which can occur with tumor patients, for example. This makes the grief process even more similar to that after the actual loss of a close loved one. Family caregivers should be informed about this phenomenon of anticipatory grief so that feelings of guilt do not develop if the thought of the death of the person with dementia or their actual death is not followed by a reaction of grief (see Case Example 43).

12.3.2 Complicated Grief Reaction

International studies show that family members do not always adapt to the loss of a loved one with dementia. Although the majority of relatives (approx. 70%) view the death of the person with dementia as a relief, about 20% of caregiving family members develop complicated feelings of grief 6 months after the death of the dementia sufferer, and 30% develop clinically relevant depressive symptoms (Schulz et al., 2006; Schulz et al., 2003). Particularly high levels of depression and burden in caregivers before the dementia sufferer's death are risk factors for the development of complicated grief and depressive symptoms. Furthermore, severe cognitive impairments of the dementia sufferer represent a predictor of increased experience of burden after the death. Even if caregiving was seen as a positive responsibility, the process of adapting to the situation of loss could be more difficult and complicated grief is more likely to develop. These possible effects should be taken into account in therapeutic work with family caregivers. Thus, confrontation with the death of dementia sufferers is an important topic in therapy. In addition, alternatives to the caregiving task can be discussed with the family members at the time of caregiving in order to prevent an "identity crisis" after the person with dementia's death.

> **Case Example 43. Anticipatory grief**
>
> The following excerpt stems from therapy with a 72-year-old wife.
>
> *Caregiver:* Lately, thoughts about the future come to mind frequently ... positive ones ... all of the things that I will be able to do ... for example, to spend several weeks at a holiday home with my friend ... to go to the theatre again ... things like that.
>
> *Therapist:* Yes, that is something very positive.
>
> *Caregiver:* Yes, sometimes I just don't know, because then I often have a guilty conscience ... then I say to myself: "Jeez, he is still here ..." You know, a couple of years ago I cried when I imagined my future without him ... but that has changed recently ... but I can't really explain it to myself ... because he's still there and actually I should be even sadder.
>
> *Therapist:* Yes, I understand what you mean. I think that because your husband has been suffering from dementia for so many years, you already started long ago to adjust yourself a bit, to a new life ... and the thought that he will one day no longer be here is no longer so threatening ... because you are actually ready to adjust to a new life. Could it be like that?
>
> *Caregiver:* Yes, somehow. I have already said goodbye to a certain extent.

Therapist: Yes, I find that quite understandable. Because it is the case with dementia that you do not lose your partner when he has died but actually much earlier, because he changes more and more and you have to say goodbye again and again ... to the conversations that you once had with one another, to the intimacy, to the shared activities.

Caregiver: Yes, none of that has existed anymore between us for a long time.

Therapist: And when that gradually became clear to you, you probably grieved heavily?

Caregiver: Yes, I fell into a hole back then.

Therapist: And now you're crawling out of it again?

Caregiver: [laughs] Yes, you could see it that way.

Therapist: And I'm sure you'll be sad too when your husband dies ...

Caregiver: Yes, I will be ... [sighs].

Therapist: But maybe it will be a little different?

Caregiver: Yes, it's also a bit of a relief for me, but also for him. It's just different than if he hadn't had the disease ... if we had lived a normal life together. But so ... yes, I probably already did say goodbye.

13
"I Need to Do It on My Own" – Support Options for Family Caregivers of Persons With Dementia

When caring for a family member with dementia, there is usually either no or very little time left for one's own needs. One reason for this is that many caregivers hardly receive or utilize support from their personal environment. Friends withdraw or show little understanding of the changed life situation. Family members are unable to help due to physical distance, their own problems, or their workload, as two caregivers explain in Example 20.

The majority of people with dementia are looked after and cared for exclusively by private individuals or family members (Schulz & Martire, 2004). This is difficult to maintain in the long term if the family caregivers do not receive additional support either financially or in terms of personnel. For this reason, there are various professional support options. The goal of professional support is to help the persons suffering from dementia, relieve the family caregivers, and promote the maintenance of care at home.

Example 20. Missing support

Caregiver: We don't want to be a burden to anyone, that is our greatest fear and concern! Our children have their own families, we cannot burden them.

Caregiver: I live near my mother. My sister benefits from not living nearby. She doesn't even call and ask if everything is going well. I understand that she can't come often due to the distance. But it puts a strain on me that she shows no interest.

She doesn't ever call me and she calls my mother once a week. I just don't think that's enough. It would help my mother a lot if she knew that there are still people who are interested in her or who are interested in her wellbeing. It would be nice if my sister asked me: "Are you okay, do you need any help?"

Despite the large number of different support options, the utilization of formal support by family caregivers is low overall (see Chapter 2). In order to encourage family caregivers to accept support, several factors need to be considered, which are addressed in this chapter.

13.1 Goals of the Module

Giving up caregiving, for example, to a nursing home, is out of the question for many family caregivers – even if they are overwhelmed. This can result in exhaustion, physical ailments, and depression. It is thus important that family caregivers receive information on support services and make use of them. The module begins with the aims of imparting to family caregivers that they have a right to receive support and showing them ways and possibilities to utilize support.

Family caregivers should be encouraged to seek and accept specific forms of help, advice and/or emotional support, based on their needs. From a therapeutic point of view, this results in the following subgoals:
- improving knowledge on and/or information about support options;
- strengthening self-help potential and self-care through actively searching for support options; and
- clarifying problems related to social support.

Box 21 contains an overview of the interventions covered in this chapter.

Box 21. Overview of the interventions

- Identifying the need for assistance
- Overcoming barriers to utilizing support
- Finding the right time
- Searching for support possibilities
- Handling difficulties with respect to the utilization

13.2 Identifying the Need for Assistance

In many cases, it is helpful in the beginning to explore the current life situation in terms of existing sources of support. The therapist can also inquire about current stressors. This sensitizes the family caregivers to the issue and encourages them to think about utilizing professional support. Especially when addressing this issue, it is important for the therapist to show appreciation for the caregivers' efforts. Examples of opening questions for analyzing the need for support are given in Questions 18.

The therapist can use techniques such as *guided discovery* or *imagination* to assess the need for support more discriminately. Furthermore, asking circular questions and changing perspective can be helpful, as the perceived need for support also depends on the point of view of the person with dementia and also other family members.

- What support would your (family member with dementia) ... wish for?
- What form of support would your ... like to have if they could choose?
- What support would your ... need in your situation?

Questions 18. Helpful opening questions

- Caregiving requires a lot of strength. Who supports you with this?
- You are doing a lot. If you ever need support, who could give it to you?
- How would they help you?
- What would they take on for you?
- With which professional support options have you already gained experience?
- What kind of support would you like in your situation?
- Imagine the perfect support option that would provide you some relief: What would it be like?

The therapy sequence in Case Example 44 demonstrates how to get started with this topic.

Many family caregivers are not used to addressing the need for support, and there is often a discrepancy between the need for and the utilization of support. Various barriers are the reason for this, which are discussed in Case Example 45.

Case Example 44. Getting started with the topic of utilization of support

The following excerpt stems from therapy with a 63-year-old caregiving wife.

Therapist: When you feel helpless and need support, who will give it to you?

Caregiver: It's difficult, I often don't know that myself. I usually try to find out everything myself. I get on my computer and search the internet.

Therapist: And are there people you would turn to if you felt helpless?

Caregiver: Actually, no, because people who don't deal with it can hardly understand what it's like. We have a friend who understands and gets along with my husband very well. I can talk to her about it. Otherwise, I don't know anyone else.

Therapist: Hmm.

Caregiver: You withdraw more and more, and it rarely happens that you talk about your experiences or what problem you are currently facing. You may get less help as a result. But there are some things that I really don't want to talk about either. That might be a mistake, but I'm not necessarily the type of person who talks about it in great detail. I'm used to dealing with a lot of things on my own.

> **Case Example 45. Difficulties with accepting help**
>
> The following excerpt stems from therapy with a 55-year-old caregiving daughter.
>
> *Caregiver:* Actually, I would also like to be able to accept help. That I can become more open. Because when there are actually people who *could* help, I still catch myself presenting our situation as being much better than it actually is, which then stalls the possibility for help.
>
> *Therapist:* You wish to show sadness and moments of weakness ...
>
> *Caregiver:* Let's say, "I'm feeling really shitty now and I'm happy that you are offering this or that." And then to take their offer.
>
> *Therapist:* Yes, yes, ok. I understand. This is an important point.
>
> *Caregiver:* When someone opens their arms and says: "It's okay to cry," you know? But ...
>
> *Therapist:* That means you wish you would allow yourself to be sad sometimes, to pay attention to your own needs, and in doing so also accept help that others offer?
>
> *Caregiver:* Yes.

13.3 Overcoming Barriers to Utilizing Support

The decision regarding whether one accepts help is a complex process (see Chapter 2). Family caregivers often experience ambivalence here, and it entails positive and negative consequences for both the caregivers and the persons with dementia. Therefore, barriers to utilizing support should be addressed and questioned. It is essential to work on individual, clearly defined barriers that can be broken through.

In principle, a distinction is made between objective and subjective obstacles (Evans & Baldwin, 1989; Gage & Kinney, 1995; Pilgram & Tschainer, 1999). However, distinguishing between objective and subjective reasons is not always easy in practice since practical reasons are often linked to personal convictions and attitudes.

Objective barriers are factors that make it difficult for family caregivers to take advantage of the offers. This includes:
- difficult organizational, financial, or situational circumstances;
- missing information about possibilities and rights, as well as contacts for help (Coe & Neufeld, 1999; Gage & Kinney, 1995); and
- problems with professional institutions and authorities.

Personal reasons or *subjective barriers* (cf. Hedtke-Becker, 1990; Pilgram & Tschainer, 1999) can be very diverse. For example, disappointing experiences with utilizing support services in the past or worries about having to give strangers a glimpse into privacy can be reasons, as the quote in Example 21 from a 57-year-old caregiving daughter shows.

Example 21. Barriers to utilizing support

> "The outpatient service usually came to bathe her at 6 a.m. and the staff often fluctuated. For me, that was more stress than support. And, actually, I don't want people that I don't know that well in our house, especially when I'm not there."

In particular, dysfunctional attitudes toward care that are associated with personal norms and values can prevent family caregivers from taking advantage of professional help (see Chapter 8). In addition to cognitive restructuring (see Chapter 8), analyzing advantages and disadvantages (according to Miller & Rollnick, 2012) is suitable for reflecting on barriers to utilizing support. The examples in Questions 19, as well as Worksheet 13-1: Should I Utilize Support? can be used to gather attitudes regarding the advantages and disadvantages of utilizing support.

Questions 19. Gathering advantages and disadvantages

> - What are the advantages of your family member being taken care of only by you?
> - What are the negative consequences of taking care of your family member on your own?
> - What arguments can be made for utilizing professional help?
> - What unfavorable or negative consequences would it have to make use of professional help?

In order to break down barriers to utilizing support, it is necessary to permanently encourage the caregivers in their plan to make use of support. At the same time, it is important to highlight and validate their previous and ongoing caregiving efforts. Case Example 46, with a caregiving daughter, illustrates this aspect.

It is helpful to encourage family caregivers repeatedly in their decision to accept support and to make it clear to them that they have a right to receive support and that accepting support can help them ensure caregiving at home for as long as possible.

13.4 Finding the Right Time for Support

Family caregivers often find it difficult to estimate their psychological burden and the resulting need for assistance. In contrast, physical impairment can often be identified more clearly. Moreover, caregiving and the energy required increases slowly over time, such that family caregivers continuously "grow into" their role and gradually take on more and more tasks. Many ask for help only when there is no other way or there is an emergency, for example, due to one's own illness. Thus, the therapist should address the caregiver's individual stress limits and possible consequences in order to find the right time at which caregivers should make use of support (see Questions 20).

Questions 20. Perceiving one's own stress limit

- Where are your limits in terms of caregiving? What would you not want to do? Who could support you then?
- If you are not able to at some point or are ill, who will take care of your family member?
- What would happen if you are not doing well at some point?

Case Example 46. Therapeutic encouragement for utilizing support

The following excerpt stems from therapy with a 64-year-old caregiving daughter.

Caregiver: Well, sometimes I think: "I can't handle this anymore."

Therapist: Yes, I believe you. What you are doing for your mother is really more than what one can manage on their own. I am concerned about your health because I understand that you are not doing well. So, it is good that you are thinking about how you can provide yourself with some relief and I think it's great that you're considering placing your mother in a day-care facility.

Caregiver: Yes! I think so too.

Therapist: Yes, that would certainly be helpful. However, I have the feeling that there are still doubts. Is that so?

Caregiver: Oh, I always feel a bit sorry for her because I know that nothing else happens in day care. I see that, of course. I say: "Have you been outside?" – "No."

Therapist: And your concern is that she will exercise less when she is there?

Caregiver: Exactly, that's my concern. That they then take everything off her shoulders and that she then ... well, deteriorates very quickly and ends up where I actually don't want her to be yet. That's just how it is. No one can convince me otherwise.

Therapist: Yes, that's possible. However, it's worth a try. Let's say it's an experiment for now, and you give it a try for 4 weeks, on a temporary basis. And if your health improves, as a result, it will be good for both of you. You will still look after her every afternoon and around the clock on the weekends as well. That will still be a lot of weight on your shoulders.

Caregiver: Right, I'll do it that way first. I know that I will do that with the day care. I know that I'll do that.

Therapist: You seem to be a little relieved now?

Caregiver: Oh [exhales deeply], I'm relieved now, that you are also recommending it to me, and that I can talk to someone about it.

Many family caregivers find it difficult to perceive their own stress limits. This is also compounded by feelings of shame, the feeling of having failed, or the fear of transferring caregiving to someone else.

For many family caregivers, imagining their own illness is also fear inducing and associated with worrying. This often leads to caregivers avoiding a solution-based confrontation with their own stress limits through thoughts like, "Everything will be fine. I just can't be absent." A solution-based confrontation with these fears and worries that is carefully guided by the therapist can increase the motivation to utilize support. Sometimes a caregiver's acute illness also provides an opportunity to talk about the future and emergency strategies, as Case Example 47 shows.

Case Example 47. Limits of caregiving: Caregiver's own illness

The following excerpt stems from therapy with a 66-year-old caregiving wife.

Caregiver: I had a bit of a cold now and had to lie down, but it had to come to this at some point. I think that so much had just come together … right?

Therapist: I can tell from your voice that you are still feeling under the weather.

Caregiver: Yes.

Therapist: Hmm.

Caregiver: But I think, as I said, that it's just mental, right? I have been thinking for over a year that the body will at one point say: "Enough!" It was just a matter of time.

Therapist: That your body is sending a signal.

Caregiver: Yes.

Therapist: That it's time to rest.

Caregiver: Yes.

Therapist: You said that a lot has come together lately.

Caregiver: Yes, all of last year. And also, through our talk, I have to say. I think about a lot of things differently now.

Therapist: Hmm.

Caregiver: So I brood about a lot and even more about the future and how long it will go well and what if it doesn't. I don't really want to have to think that far ahead. I'm a little scared of that, I have to say. I only became aware of that through our talks.

Therapist: Okay. Mm-hmm. So the talks, they set something in motion. Right?

Caregiver: Yes.

Therapist: What else was going through your mind?

Caregiver: Yes, actually, what I have managed and had to do over the last year and had to consider, and yes. It's also a lot of running around. Also dealing with health insurance companies. Stuff like that.

Therapist: Yes.

Caregiver: I have to do everything on my own here. I can't delegate anything.

Therapist: You have no support; you do everything by yourself.

Caregiver: Yes.

Therapist: Well, that's a lot, what you're doing. And then to first realize everything that your husband's illness entails – everything that you have to do alone, where you have to make decisions on your own, paths that you have to go alone. Well, you can quickly reach your limit.

Caregiver: Yes, I have to take care of everything.

Therapist: Yes. And you probably often feel left alone and burdened, right?

Caregiver: Yes, exactly.

Therapist: You said that our talks made you brood. Before that, you didn't really want to think about what would come to you.

Caregiver: I can't really think about it like that. So you think about it, but it's like ... Now I definitely don't want to have to commit myself to anything specific.

Therapist: What do you mean by "anything specific?"

Caregiver: If someone came now and would say something about a nursing home and would take him away ... well, I'm scared of that. I must say. All of this only gradually became clear to me when I became sick now. And then you think about it. You sleep during the day, and then you are rested at night [laughs].

Therapist: And your mind, it's working at night.

Caregiver: And the mind is working and working and working. And that's when I actually first noticed that I couldn't stop it.

Therapist: So when you have a chance to rest.

Caregiver: You don't get to rest at all.

Therapist: Well, I mean, when you get to rest physically, you first notice then everything that is working internally, how much you do for your husband and what happens when you're absent.

Caregiver: Yes, as I said, in the past few days, I really had time to think about a lot and what is to come. One doesn't really want to know all of it, right?

Therapist: So, I think it has both sides, right? On the one hand, it is certainly not so bad if you don't always think about it, because it also takes energy and makes you sad and ... hmm and you have to somehow still function in everyday life. And the other side is, I believe, from the experiences we also have with other family caregivers, is that's also – I would say it is painful to deal with, but on the other side it is good to prepare for what is to come. Not to ignore it entirely, but to explore your own feelings and to be prepared.

Caregiver: Yes, I can't ignore it anyway.

Therapist: Yes.

It is also helpful to consider various emergency strategies. Questions 21 contains helpful examples.

Questions 21. Emergency strategies

- Who will take care of them if you are prevented from doing so at short notice, e.g., for a day?
- What happens if you are absent for more than a week?
- What happens if you need help yourself?
- What happens to your ... in an emergency?

The answers to these questions can result in an emergency plan. In addition to the action steps, the emergency plan contains the most important contact addresses and telephone numbers (see Worksheet 13-2: Emergency Plan). Developing support measures in an assumed emergency situation helps to increase the willingness to accept support even if an emergency does not occur.

Case Example 48 illustrates how the subject of an emergency situation can be discussed with the caregivers.

> **Case Example 48. Precautions in case of an emergency**
>
> The following excerpt stems from therapy with a 76-year-old caregiving wife.
>
> *Therapist:* For today we had decided to discuss an emergency plan in the event that you become ill for a long time yourself and have to temporarily give caregiving to someone else.
>
> *Caregiver:* Yes, although I don't really want to think about it. But because of my hip problems, I think it makes a lot of sense.
>
> *Therapist:* Yes, it definitely does. Because then you will have prepared for an emergency.
>
> *Caregiver:* Yes, and I still hope that I don't have to take it out of the drawer and use it.
>
> *Therapist:* Right, and if you should ever need it, you will know where it is.
>
> *Caregiver:* Yes, exactly, that is good.
>
> *Therapist:* It would be good if we clarified the "what, who, where, and how." By what, I mean the question "What should happen in an emergency situation?" that is, when you can no longer take care of your husband. And who should help you then?
>
> *Caregiver:* Well, it would be an emergency if I had to go to the hospital because of my hip joint. But then both of my daughters would step in. They would take him in at first. But that's only possible for a short time, they both work. After that, he would have to go to a facility.
>
> *Therapist:* Ah yes, that's great that your daughters support you. Then what exactly should your daughters do?
>
> *Caregiver:* Yes, I can rely on both of them. They would then have to organize a place for short-term care.
>
> *Therapist:* Have you already used that before?
>
> *Caregiver:* No, but I know from another caregiving wife that it works.
>
> *Therapist:* Ah yes, do you know the address and how to organize it?
>
> *Caregiver:* No, but I could ask her about that.
>
> *Therapist:* Yes, that would be very good. She may also be able to give you tips so that you can clarify "where and how" your husband should be looked after in case of an emergency. Could you imagine speaking with her about it before our next phone call?
>
> *Caregiver:* Yes, I can definitely do that.
>
> *Therapist:* Perhaps you could then write down the address and telephone numbers for your daughters on an emergency plan.
>
> *Caregiver:* Yes, that's a good idea. I will do that. I will also discuss this with my daughters.

13.5 Searching for Support Options

If family caregivers signal a need for support and possible related obstacles have already been discussed, it is advisable to accelerate the active search for support. With the increasing need for help, professional support gains importance, which is why it is recommended to search for professional support options in addition to private ones. Since many family caregivers are not sufficiently informed about existing support options, it may be necessary as a first step to inform them that several support options exist from which they can choose. The therapist can also ask about specific support options in order to uncover possible information deficits (see Questions 22).

Questions 22. Support options

- Do you know about the different care options for people with dementia? Which do you know?
- Which counseling and support services are available in your region?

Since the support options vary greatly from region to region, especially between rural and urban regions, the therapist should get an overview of possible support services in advance. Various brochures and internet portals, for example from regional Alzheimer's Societies, can be used. Family caregivers should also be encouraged to independently obtain information about support options. In doing so, the caregivers' self-efficacy is strengthened and their conscious decision for accepting support is encouraged. Moreover, by having this knowledge, family caregivers can make use of support options after the therapy sessions have been concluded.

The technique of problem solving can be used to support the process of searching for support services, which also encourages the caregivers' problem-solving competence. It is important that the problem-solving process in terms of the appropriateness of the support options is always evaluated together with the family caregivers (see also Chapter 11).

Family caregiver self-help groups represent an important source for support, also in terms of a social resource. They offer the opportunity to exchange ideas with other affected individuals. Guided groups are groups that are led by an expert (e.g., a social worker) who is very familiar with the problems and burdens of caregivers and who can provide additional information.

Family caregiver self-help groups can offer information or advice and thus encourage a change in how the situation is handled, for example by offering opportunities for instrumental support such as care services, as well as behavioral strategies that strengthen or impart coping skills or that improve emotional well-being through stress management techniques (Senelick, 2016). This is summarized in Table 6.

Other offers can promote networking among family caregivers, such as dance or music events, cafés, senior citizen trips, supervised vacations, attending lectures and events on the subject of dementia, and working/volunteering in associations.

In the caregivers' residential area, contact with friends and neighbors should be encouraged. As a result, participation in active life can be partially retained for the persons with dementia and their caregivers. Removing the taboo on dementia and openly dealing with the disease among friends and acquaintances also contributes to this. In particular, the withdrawal from social life by many family caregivers should be addressed, as shown in Example 22.

Example 22. Withdrawal due to dementia

> *Caregiver:* Of course, friends don't understand that you limit your life in such a way. It is fun to talk to them, but the worries and needs are different. As a result, all of it is relatively superficial for me. The conversations are no longer so important, we used to be on the same level, and today I'm in a completely different life situation. My point of view has changed. And I can't expect everyone else to understand that. We have therefore withdrawn ourselves a bit.

From the multitude of options mentioned, it is advisable to select and try out those that are tailored to the family caregiver's individual wishes and personality. The possibility of no longer making use of an option or exchanging one option for another should also be emphasized. The search for suitable support should be understood as a process that changes according to the caregiver's phase of life and stage in the caregiving process. In Case Example 49, a caregiver reports on a talk with an employee of a nursing service.

Table 6. Support for family caregivers

Professional support options	
Medical and psychological support	General practitioner care and specialists (neurology, psychiatry), dementia-specific facilities (e.g., memory clinics), psychotherapy for family caregivers
Counselling and information	Regional Alzheimer's societies, regional consultation centers, care support points, family caregiver and self-help groups, caregiving counselors, telephone counseling, email counseling, internet, training for caregivers, publications, magazines and information brochures, self-help contact points

13.6 Difficulties Regarding Utilization of Support

13.6.1 Asking for Help

Asking for help and support is difficult for most family caregivers, but especially for caregiving wives. On the one hand, they do not want to be a burden to anyone and, on the other hand, they do not want to admit that they need help. Feelings of shame and guilt (e.g., admitting to feeling overwhelmed) can also make this step more difficult. The therapy excerpt in Case Example 50 illustrates asking family members for support, discussed with a caregiving wife. It shows how difficult it is for the caregiving wife to ask her daughters for support.

Role-playing can be suitable to prepare situations in which the caregivers wish to ask for a specific form of help. The therapy excerpt in Case Example 51 illustrates this with a caregiving daughter asking her sister for help.

Case Example 49. Positive consequences of using professional support

The following excerpt stems from therapy with a 64-year-old caregiving daughter.

Caregiver: And then she said: "How can we arrange an overnight stay so that you can have a night off sometime? I have an idea. I would stay overnight. Ms. L., could you imagine that?" She gave a friendly smile, and I asked: "Yes, but what are you doing on this specific night?" – "Yes, I could then sit here in the living room."

I thought: "*Wow!*" then I got on the computer and looked up hotels and bed and breakfasts in the area and thought: "What will I do? Do I go there in the evening and get a room, go into the tub and sleep there and have breakfast, and then come back, or do I buy fresh bread and then come back?" And then a bit of a sense of reality came back again, and I thought: "No, maybe you have to stay at home for the first night. They might also have some questions, or they might be unable to find something, or maybe something else." But yes, my imagination got wings right away [laughs].

But I was so ... overwhelmed by the offer that I burst into tears [starts to cry] and said to the good woman: "I find it so great how you, with your nursing service, how it ... that it works in a personal way." Then she hugged me and said: "You know, that is also the advantage of a very small nursing service that you can respond to the wishes of the patients much more individually." I hope that we can continue to do it this way for a long time.

Therapist: That is great. That you have a night to look forward to and then sleep in a bed and breakfast or meet up with a friend. That sounds really wonderful.

Caregiver: To be out of the cage suddenly. A door from the cage opens. Sometimes I feel like I'm in a cage.

Case Example 50. Asking family members for support

The following excerpt stems from therapy with an 84-year-old caregiving wife.

Caregiver: So, I'll just ask them [the children] about it. If they do it, that'll be good. If they don't do it, that'll be good too. Then I can make different arrangements.

Therapist: Oh, I think that's great!

Caregiver: I'll just bring it up with them.

Therapist: How did you come to this decision now to ask your children for help? You didn't dare to do that 2 weeks ago.

Caregiver: I thought: "Now first see that we have a little more contact again and see whether they come to us on their own," or if I have to say again "Hey, listen, you haven't been around for 4 weeks, and it's time ..." And then it actually occurred to me that I have nothing to lose, so to speak. At the moment, my husband no longer misses his children.

Therapist: You mentioned that once, yes.

Caregiver: And it won't hurt him, and I can manage without them if they don't want to help. That's not the problem for me either. Which means, I can actually just say to them: "Are you going to help or not?"

Therapist: You could be disappointed, couldn't you?

Caregiver: Yes, sure, I would be disappointed. But then I would also know where I stand.

Therapist: And that's what's predominant, right? That you just have clarity and know what you can and cannot expect.

Caregiver: Exactly.

Therapist: I think that's excellent. Yes, that you just want to ask again. Great!

Caregiver: Maybe I just have to talk to my children clearly and directly. Maybe they have no idea otherwise, I don't know.

Therapist: Yes, yes, I think so. You had already mentioned that, that when you ask someone, they can always still say "yes" or "no." You still have to ask the question first. And then you can take a step back and see where you stand and think about it. I'm looking forward to how it turns out, Ms. A.

Caregiver: Me too [laughs].

Case Example 51. Role-playing: Asking family members for support

The following excerpt stems from therapy with a 51-year-old caregiving daughter.

Caregiver: I was really angry with my sister. I understand that she has young children, but she doesn't tend to my mother at all – I have to deal with everything. That irritates me.

Therapist: I can understand that well. Last time we discussed that you would talk to her when you see her again.

Caregiver: Yes, but mom was there the whole time, and then we went out to eat too, so I didn't want to bring it up. It certainly would have dampened the mood.

Therapist: Yes, that's understandable.

Caregiver: Well, I don't know what to say to her either. Should I say, for example, "I want you to visit mom once a week." Then she'll react snottily and there'll be silence for the time being.

Therapist: What do you think about us role-playing the situation and seeing how the conversation goes?

Caregiver: I don't know, role-playing isn't really my thing.

Therapist: Yes, most people find it difficult. Most importantly, it's not so easy to ask your sister for support. That's why I think role-playing would be very good, we could try it out. I'll be your sister, and you approach me, okay? When and where would you approach her?

Caregiver: Preferably on the phone, otherwise mom is always there.

Therapist: Okay, what do you want to ask of her? What do you need support with?

Caregiver: I want her to tend to mom more, and not just when I say something.

Therapist: Can you formulate that again in specific terms?

Caregiver: I actually want her to come by once a week. She doesn't have to do anything, just come for a short visit.

Therapist: Okay, what exactly should she do?

Caregiver: It would be nice if she came by on Thursday, for an hour or so. I could then go shopping in peace.

Therapist: Okay, you would ask her. What would you have to watch out for when you ask her to do that?

Caregiver: I have to be careful not to get upset, otherwise we'll quickly end up in an argument, and then nothing works anymore.

Therapist: Yes, that's possible; some caregivers experience this. What could you do to ensure that you don't get upset on the phone?

Caregiver: Yes, I don't know either. I know her, I know that nothing comes from her end.

Therapist: That means that you hardly have any expectations of her?

Caregiver: Yes, hardly.

Therapist: What could you say to yourself to calm yourself down during the conversation?

Caregiver: Well, I could say to myself: Actually, it's not that important that she comes. I have to do everything by myself anyway. Then she won't see her mother, but that has nothing to do with me. Until now, I've managed everything on my own.

Therapist: Okay, that would create a little distance?

Caregiver: Yes, maybe.

Therapist: Okay, then let's try it.

Caregiver: Well, alright.

Therapist: Okay. You start. Ring, ring!

Caregiver: Hello, M. [sister's first name], I wanted to get in touch. How's D. [caregiver's nephew] doing? I haven't seen him in a while.

Therapist: We're doing well, but there's a lot to do, you know.

Caregiver: Yes, same here. Hey, I wanted to ask if you can come visit Mom this week, preferably with D., Mom is always so happy to see him. Perhaps on Thursday?

Therapist: Yes, I would like to, but this week I really can't. There's just too much going on.

Caregiver: It's also your mother. You could at least visit her.

Therapist: Yes, maybe next week.

Caregiver: Could you come next Thursday? I would like to go shopping on Thursday. Mom and I will be home starting at 4:30 p.m.

Therapist: I have a lot to do, but if you need me, I can arrange it.

Caregiver: Yes, that would be nice. Can I count on you?

Therapist: I'll write it down.

Caregiver: Great, see you Thursday.

Therapist: Okay. We'll stop here. How was that for you?

Caregiver: Yes, quite realistic and I noticed that I actually don't like to ask her and I was quickly upset when she said no at first.

Therapist: Yes, asking for support is difficult for most caregivers, but it is very important because without support it is immensely difficult to provide care over a long period of time. And your sister may not even know how much you do for your mother every day and that you would like some support.

Caregiver: I think so too.

Therapist: That's why it's very important that you ask your sister about it directly. How did you feel doing it?

Caregiver: Well, a little weird. I don't usually ask her so directly. I think she should notice it on her own.

Therapist: Yes, that would be nice. I found it good – in my role as your sister that you directly asked me about Thursday. Then I knew exactly what I was supposed to do and I could then make arrangements.

Caregiver: Yes, but she also has a small family, and with two small children it's also not easy. She probably wouldn't have time anyway.

Therapist: Yes, she may react differently, we don't know that. How about you try it out with your sister on the phone before our next session?

Caregiver: Yes, I'll do that. I'll at least ask her directly.

Therapist: I find that great. I know that it's not easy for you.

The example shows that the caregiver's sister does not want to take care of the mother due to her own burdens. Therefore, the therapist worked with the caregiver to accept this fact and at the same time to look for professional support options.

13.6.2 Working With Professional Services

When working with professional care services, difficulties may arise due to caregivers' fears and concerns, for example, "I don't want to have strangers in my house all the time," as well as due to insecurities and feelings of guilt or shame, for example, "Am I permitted to put him in day care at all?" "I must be a bad wife. I'm not doing enough." These thoughts should be processed using cognitive techniques. On the other hand, the person suffering from dementia can refuse the offer of support, as Example 23 illustrates.

Example 23. Rejection of a support offer by the care recipient

> *Caregiver:* My husband had told me in a very quiet moment that he thinks it's terrible in day care, because it's so boring there, and that he's the only one who has everything in sight, everyone else had stepped away a bit, and he doesn't know what to do with himself there. And then my guilty conscience came back immediately. This feeling was very intense, and I thought: Oh, I've given him away. Should I take him out of there and put him somewhere else?

Difficulties often result, however, from information deficits, organizational problems (e.g., change of nursing staff), caregivers' specific quality standards (e.g., duration of the care service too short), as well as a lack of flexibility of the offers (e.g., unfavorable time of care). These problems require contact or a discussion with the professional service. Finding alternative services can also be helpful. Case Example 52 illustrates this.

In the event of setbacks and negative experiences regarding support services, the therapist can provide emotional support and discuss alternative options or conflict resolutions. Questions 23 gives helpful examples that can be worked out in advance, to prevent conflicts with professional services.

Questions 23. Prepare oneself on using professional services

> - How do you feel about the idea of using … [a nursing service]?
> - What should you be prepared for? What will be different?
> - What feelings arise when you imagine yourself being supported by a professional nurse?

Finally, Worksheet 13-3: Which Support Is Suitable for My Situation? can be filled out with the family caregivers, where all possible support offers can be written down once again.

13.6.3 Family Caregivers Expect Support From the Therapist Regarding Legal and Organizational Questions

Every now and then, family caregivers may seek psychotherapeutic support because they are hoping for help in dealing with authorities or insurance companies. In such cases, it is important to explain to the family caregivers that such support cannot be part of psychotherapy, but that specific advisory centers (e.g., care advisors, care service centers) are responsible for these issues. However, in terms of these topics, the therapy sessions can be used, for example, to find ways in which the family caregivers can deal constructively with decisions made by authorities and other institutions.

> **Case Example 52. The caregiver's requirements**
>
> The following excerpt stems from therapy with a 72-year-old caregiving wife.
>
> *Caregiver:* I once put him in short-term care in spring and, when I picked him up, I went in – it was noon – the door to the room was open, the heater was off, outside it was very cold. The room and my husband were both freezing cold. He had three new injuries on his legs. They should nurse him only in his room, and not around the whole group, because I know that he'll get upset and kick his legs around. That's stressful for my husband. And an old person, especially with dementia, no longer knows what's going on around them. This is a threat to him, he gets upset. I don't want him to be completely confused when he gets back. And that's how it turned out. And we know how the situation is with nursing staff. Ever since I saw that – him sitting in the cold – well he could get pneumonia.
>
> *Therapist:* You were not satisfied with the quality of care in short-term care. You were very upset about that.
>
> *Caregiver:* Yes, yes, he always used to tell me that he didn't like it that much in the home. But I said: "Look, I want to go on vacation too, and then you can have contact with other people." What did I not say is that I thought: "Well okay, he'll survive for the time being and then you'll be able to have vacation" and then I went somewhere for 8 days.
>
> *Therapist:* That sounds good. It is also very important that you took some time off. Also a nurse doesn't work around the clock without ever taking a vacation.
>
> *Caregiver:* Yes, but I'm not putting him in that short-term care again.
>
> *Therapist:* Okay, you weren't happy with that. Have you ever thought about alternatives?
>
> *Caregiver:* Well, there aren't that many here.
>
> *Therapist:* Have you ever looked at other short-term care facilities?
>
> *Caregiver:* No.
>
> *Therapist:* There are very different ones. Perhaps another facility will suit your needs better? What would a facility need to have so that you could use it without having a guilty conscience?
>
> *Caregiver:* Well, it would have to be a small facility and they would also have to be familiar with people suffering from dementia.
>
> *Therapist:* Could you ask your Alzheimer's Society about where short-term care facilities are located in your area that also specialize in people with dementia before our next session?
>
> *Caregiver:* Yes, I can do that.

14 Nursing-Home Placement – When the Limits of Home Care Have Been Reached

Many people suffering from dementia and their caregivers favor care at home. Therefore, it is generally the goal to support their wish for home care. Nevertheless, there are situations in which care at home is no longer possible, for example if the family caregivers reach their psychological and/or physical limits related to the caregiving situation or if the person with dementia can no longer be adequately cared for at home (Hähnel et al., 2023). Once home-care limits have been reached, it is reasonable for the caregivers to look into alternatives (see Example 24).

Example 24. When is the right time for Nursing-Home Placement?

Therapist: You know, I think it's really wonderful that you say, "Actually, it is a wish of me to care for her myself until the end." Of course, we also discuss with a large number of family caregivers the question of when it is no longer possible. "Can this point come up at some point in time?" And the time when it comes is very different for each individual.

Caregiver: When is the point? Yes, sometimes I think: "How long do you want to wait until we both fall down?" If she can no longer hold herself up and falls, I inevitably fall with her, because I will no longer be able to hold her up either. Then I often think: "Do you want to wait until someone has fallen so bad that they're in a wheelchair? How long do you want to wait now?" And if something does happen, then I would blame myself again and think: "Why didn't you put her in a home beforehand?"

14.1 Goals of the Module

The aim of the module is to look into alternatives to home care and to develop strategies for this transition. In order to discuss alternatives to home care with family caregivers, their current stress situation should first be addressed. Based on this, attitudes and barriers regarding alternatives can be reflected on, and assistance is given. Psychoeducation, cognitive techniques, and problem-solving strategies are hereby helpful interventions. Box 22 contains an overview of the interventions covered in this chapter.

Box 22. Overview of the interventions

- Decision-making factors
- Support in decision making
- Dealing with an emergency situation
- Encouraging the processing and acceptance of the decision
- Therapeutic procedure for dealing with intolerable caregiving situations

14.2 Decision-Making Factors

In advance, the therapist should work out current stresses and motives that have led the family caregivers to consider nursing-home care. Sometimes it may be necessary for the therapist to initiate discussion of this issue, even if the family caregivers have not considered it. This applies in particular in the event that home care can no longer be adequately guaranteed due to excessive demands, health risks, or problems in taking care of the person with dementia.

Reasons for nursing-home care are most notably health problems of the family caregivers, an increase in caregiving burden, and an associated overstrain for the caregivers. Further reasons for nursing-home care are:

- increasing deterioration of the person with dementia's health;
- an increase in the need for care (e.g., due to the person with dementia being bedridden);

- changes in behavior or an increase in problem behaviors, e.g., aggressive behavior;
- caregivers' doubts about being able to continue providing care in the future;
- lack of caregiving assistance, e.g., in the case of severe care dependency;
- lack of caregiving assistance at night, e.g., in the case of disturbed night–day rhythm;
- insufficient functionality or safety in the person with dementia's household;
- the changed life situation of the caregiver, e.g., change of place of employment;
- incompatibility between work and caregiving; and
- family reasons, e.g., separation.

The decision-making process regarding nursing-home care is very complex and usually goes through different phases (Naleppa, 1996). The decision-making factors relate to the person with dementia (e.g., degree of autonomy and ability to make their own decisions), to the caregivers (e.g., health status, feelings, attitudes, appraisal of the caregiving role, caregiving motivation), as well as to the context of the caregiving situation and aspects of the family dynamics. The terms of care should therefore be discussed with the caregivers with respect to their complexity and ambivalence.

14.2.1 Encouraging Caregivers to Reflect on Their Stress Limits

The temporal perspectives of caregiving should be discussed with the caregivers, that is, how long care at home can be provided, under which conditions they would like to end caregiving, and which alternatives could be considered (e.g., professional support for care at home). This can help the caregivers to be able to judge their own stress limits better and to discuss and plan the transfer of caregiving responsibilities openly.

In Case Example 53, the therapist encourages the caregiver to reflect on her stress limits. Sometimes it may also be necessary to confront the caregiver directly about the consequences of continuing home care.

In Case Example 54, it becomes clear that the caregiver's health is usually an important reason for placing the family member with dementia in a nursing home. However, this aspect is often underestimated by caregivers and should thus be explored precisely.

14.2.2 Feelings of Guilt and Fear of Making the Wrong Decision

In addition to the well-being of the caregivers and the person with dementia, the available resources (e.g., financial resources, support) and the general conditions (e.g., availability and quality of the nursing home), the caregivers' appraisal of the situation, the quality of the relationship, and the caregivers' feelings (such as anger, fury, helplessness) are also important key factors regarding nursing-home placement. When caregivers grapple with the transition to nursing-home care, this is not only associated with feelings of being overwhelmed, helplessness, and the desire for relief but also with feelings of

---

Case Example 53. Raising awareness of stress limits

The following excerpt stems from therapy with a 60-year-old caregiving wife.

Therapist: "If I can't manage it anymore, then maybe a nursing home is necessary." What does that mean? If you can't manage it anymore, how would you notice that?

Caregiver: Well, I'll either go crazy [laugh] or I'll kill him or – no. I won't do that. That's nonsense! But ... uh ... I think it definitely depends on the situation, although you really have to be honest with yourself, "This isn't working anymore."

Therapist: You said: "Or I'll kill him." I think there's a lot to it, specifically: "Where are my limits?" And that also applies to the question of when it's no longer good for your husband. How far does it have to go? You said: "I'll go crazy" – that would be – "when I can't take it anymore." So, if that's how you define it, I would say: "Oh, no, the line has to be drawn much earlier, because then it's too late."

Caregiver: Then it's too late. That's right.

Therapist: Before you kill him – so to speak – now, right? – it's probably better to see *sooner* at which point you're not good for your husband anymore.

Case Example 54. The caregiver's health problems

The following excerpt stems from therapy with an 86-year-old caregiving wife.

Caregiver: I haven't been well in the past few weeks. My blood pressure is not good, neither is my blood sugar. My family doctor wanted to refer me to a clinic, but that's not possible. How could it be possible? Who's going to take care of my husband then?

Therapist: Yes, that doesn't sound good. What did your doctor say about your health?

Caregiver: Well, she said that I urgently need a little more rest. My blood pressure is way too high. She said something has to change soon.

Therapist: Ah yes, and how do you see it?

Caregiver: Well, I think so too. I'm not even able to relax that much at night. If I could sleep through a few nights again, that would be good. Then my blood pressure would be better. And if I could go swimming again, that would be good for me too. And when I think that I'll be 87 in July. You already notice a few aches and pains.

Therapist: Yes, I think you're doing a tremendous amount every day. You care for your husband around the clock, even though your own health is not good. In contrast to professional caregivers, you have no vacation, no substitution, and no after-work hours, and you will be 87 years old in July. So, what you do for your husband is really amazing. That's why I'm worried about you, and your health. I wonder how long you can still provide care. And what if you get seriously ill?

Caregiver: Yes, I don't really want to think about that, but I guess I have to. I just haven't had the heart to put him in a home. When you've been together for as long as we have, you can't even imagine being apart. How should I tell him that? And so far, it has still worked out somehow.

Therapist: Yes, it has been fine at home so far. Nevertheless, I notice that your health is currently very bad. That's what I'm worried about. What could you possibly change so that you can regain your strength?

Caregiver: Oh, I also notice that something has to change because of my blood pressure. Even if I would like it to be different, it can't really go on like this anymore.

Therapist: Yes, even if you would like it to be different, now is definitely a good time to talk about new ways for caregiving.

Caregiver: For us, new ways means a nursing home. Because day care would not relieve me.

Therapist: Yes, that is understandable. Because your husband needs care around the clock, and you can't do that alone at home without having health-related consequences for yourself.

Caregiver: Yes, that's true. I just simply can't anymore.

guilt, shame, and grief. It is important to support the caregivers in recognizing and dealing with the ambivalence of their feelings, thoughts, and behavior with regard to home care. Clarifying the decision-making factors helps family caregivers to gain more clarity in the complex judgment process and makes it easier to make a conscious decision for or against nursing-home care (see Case Example 55).

14.2.3 Information on Institutional Care

Existing prejudices about care facilities may be why many caregivers hardly find out about full nursing-home care or only when they need it urgently. In addition, nursing-home care is often viewed by relatives as inadequate. This makes it difficult for them to consider nursing homes as an alternative to home care, as Example 25 illustrates.

Case Example 55. Feelings of guilt and fear of responsibility

The following excerpt stems from therapy with 53-year-old caregiving daughter.

Therapist: I believe that this has a function that you – I'll just put it this way – use your family as an excuse a little for the nursing-home placement.

Caregiver: Yes, that can be.

Therapist: Do you have any idea why you are doing this? Why is this important to you?

Caregiver: [Exhales] Well ok, it may be that I … yes, that I have certain feelings of guilt about giving him away and then just want to share the decision with my family so that my feelings of guilt are not so strong. That may be.

Therapist: Mm-hmm. We had the topic "fear of making the wrong decision." And that you would like to share the responsibility that you have. So, in the end you are the one making the decision. You decide. And I think that makes you afraid of wanting to decide that on your own. And that's why you might feel better when you say: "Well, actually the others decided that for me."

Caregiver: Yes. Yes, that can be.

Therapist: And that provides inner relief.

Caregiver: Yes.

Therapist: What could help you to really … really take responsibility for yourself and say: "I've made that decision now?"

Example 25. Concerns about nursing home care

> *Caregiver:* I'm scared because one hears a lot of bad things about nursing homes. I am afraid that she will not be looked after in the same way as she is looked after by me. Basically, she is in tune with me. Above all, everything is unfamiliar to her there, especially at night – these are things that I'm still a little afraid of. She certainly won't be engaged as much there as she is here with me. I am afraid that she will then deteriorate more quickly and her condition will worsen. And when I see her sitting here in the living room and she looks out the window into our garden and is enjoying it, then I say to myself: "Stop, stop. Try again at home."

By providing family caregivers with information about care in a nursing home and asking them to obtain information themselves, a decision for or against nursing-home placement in a well-founded manner can be prepared.

Caregivers should be encouraged by the therapist to obtain information; for instance, from print media such as magazines and brochures as well as from the internet and friends and relatives. It can also be helpful to make contact with nursing homes, health insurance companies, physicians, and occupational therapists. In addition, communicating and exchanging experiences with other affected persons can be useful, for example in a family caregiver self-help group. Visiting a nursing home for information events or open houses is also recommended. In addition, Worksheet 14-1: What Should Be Considered When Choosing a Nursing Home? (translated and modified from the Deutsche Alzheimer Gesellschaft e.V. Selbsthilfe Demenz [German Alzheimer Society, self-help dementia], 2019) can be helpful – see Appendix or see booklet "Selecting and Moving into a Care Home" (Alzheimer's Society UK, 2018).

Nevertheless, most family caregivers find it difficult to occupy themselves with searching for information, as Case Example 56 illustrates.

In summary, it is important to encourage and support the family caregivers to obtain as much information as possible from different sources on the subject of institutional care in order to be well prepared in an emergency, even if dealing with the topic leads to stressful feelings such as guilt and grief.

> **Case Example 56. Informing oneself about a nursing home**
>
> The following excerpt stems from therapy with a 66-year-old caregiving daughter.
>
> *Therapist:* Did you inform yourself about nursing homes in your area, as we had discussed last time?
>
> *Caregiver:* Well, I've already learned a lot about the homes in F. One is especially excellent for people with dementia. And that would probably be the first choice for me. But, of course, there are long waiting lists, and somehow ... I still hesitate to put him on a waiting list, I have to say that in all honestly. That's another point for me. I don't want to yet.
>
> *Therapist:* I can understand that. This surely triggers uncomfortable feelings in you. Did you go and look at the home?
>
> *Caregiver:* No, I only know about it from hearsay, from different people.
>
> *Therapist:* What is stopping you from going and looking at it?
>
> *Caregiver:* Yes. Because I still have the thought in the back of my mind of whether it wouldn't be possible to make it at home with even more help. Because the care is better at home. But in the meantime, without my father's knowledge, I first talked to my brother about the fact that we would have to organize something in the event of an emergency, in case it no longer works at home.
>
> *Therapist:* Yes, so it would be a good idea to find out about a home in advance. That would have the advantage that you would already be well informed in case your father has to move to a home at short notice. You would then already know the home, possibly also some of the nursing staff. You would know what the rooms look like, and you could think beforehand about how you want to design the room for your father so that he feels comfortable there.
>
> *Caregiver:* Yes, that's true.
>
> *Therapist:* What else do you need or want to know about the home?
>
> *Caregiver:* Well. Who still lives there. Whether the nurses also go for a walk with the people. How the food is. Which activities are available.
>
> *Therapist:* So you have very specific questions that you could clarify on site. It would be best if you got an impression of the home for yourself. In your folder, you can also find an information sheet on what to consider when choosing a nursing home. Perhaps additional questions will arise that you can ask.

14.3 Support in Decision Making

In addition to imparting knowledge and information, cognitive restructuring methods can be used in assisting family caregivers in the decision-making process, with the following objectives:
- reflecting on the positive and negative aspects as well as consequences of nursing home care; and
- developing realistic expectations regarding nursing home care.

14.3.1 Reflecting on the Positive and Negative Aspects As Well As Consequences of Nursing Home Care

The decision-making process can be made easier if family caregivers precisely reflect on and consider reasons against nursing-home placement and relief through nursing-home placement. The therapist should encourage family caregivers to state both positive and negative aspects of nursing-home placement. A clear distinction between nursing tasks and emotional care can be worked out. Thus, for many family caregivers, the realization that they can possibly be there much more for the person with dementia through placing them in a nursing home is par-

> **Case Example 57. Assisted living is to be equated with "not taking care anymore"**
>
> The following excerpt stems from therapy with a 64-year-old caregiving wife.
>
> *Therapist:* You had equated assisted living with being kicked out. Kicking out and living in, as it is now, are two poles. And I'm quite sure that there is a lot in between. For example, one can have their family members in assisted living and still have a lot of contact with them and be there for them. It's not either/or. That doesn't mean: "I'll push him into the home and really let go and not care about him anymore."
>
> *Caregiver:* No, for God's sake [laughing].
>
> *Therapist:* So, here, there is very, very much in between.
>
> *Caregiver:* Mm-hmm. I just simply can't completely see what it's like there.
>
> *Therapist:* I had sessions with a daughter who was caring for her mother. At the beginning of the sessions, the mother was still at home. The conflict was there from the start. The thought of putting her in a home was associated with a guilty conscience. But she got to the point where she said: "But actually, I can't take this anymore." By now, the mother lives in the home. And the daughter is there 3 hours a day. She drives there, makes tea, they have a nice park. ... The nice quality time they have there together – how much is that? Three hours. Ok. How much was it before? If we don't include the time spent cleaning, cooking, and personal hygiene, but rather the time where they really did something nice together. Well, in the end, the nursing work was so much that there might have only been an hour left for something nice. But now the daughter has 3 hours with her mother, in the park, walking, chatting, playing, and looking at photos and so on. So that's what I mean, there is a lot in between. How are you now?
>
> *Caregiver:* It's like a glimmer of hope right now [laughing].
>
> *Therapist:* What are you thinking?
>
> *Caregiver:* I'm just thinking a little bit about what it would be like if I did, you know? If I dare to take this step.

> **Case Example 58. Reality check**
>
> The following excerpt stems from therapy with a 71-year-old caregiving wife.
>
> *Therapist:* You want your husband to be doing well in the nursing home, and you want that with all your heart, and you are very alert. You give everything, you are doing everything that you can to prepare for the transition properly. You inform the nursing staff there, and you have drawn up a list, so you do everything you can to ensure that it is implemented there. And yet I believe that you have a pretty high standard of how your husband is supposed to be cared for there. Maybe it helps to compare every once in a while: How was it actually at home? For example, you said that you found it sad that your husband sat there alone when guests came over or that it is important to you that your husband goes outside. My aim is to put that into perspective again. That is important to you, of course, but in the winter months, it was not possible to do that at home either. So, do a reality check between your standards and what is even possible. Yes? Your standards have probably always remained the same. They were already so high when your husband still lived with you, but you could not always live up to them either. You had to go to work, your husband struggled to use the stairs, there were just things that were the way they were such that reaching the optimum was not always possible. But that's life.
>
> *Caregiver:* Mm-hmm.
>
> *Therapist:* And ... now your husband is in the nursing home, and you continue to measure with these standards that are too high. That's why I recommend you do a reality check every now and then: What is realistic, and what were we even able to implement at home? And while, on the one hand, certain things may not be done in the same way as they were at home, on the other hand, there may be other things that were not possible at home.

ticularly beneficial for the decision-making process. This differentiation between nursing activities in the sense of helping with activities of daily living (such as getting dressed, bathing) and more affective, emotional care is illustrated in Case Example 57. In this case example, the supposedly negative aspects of nursing-home care are more likely to be classified as dysfunctional thoughts and are therefore disputed as dysfunctional "black-and-white" thinking.

14.3.2 Working out Realistic Expectations Regarding Nursing-Home Care

Realistic expectations regarding the care of the person with dementia should be discussed and critically questioned both before and during the transition to the nursing home, as illustrated in Case Example 58.

Additionally, dealing with doubts that often arise after the decision to place the person with dementia in a nursing home should be addressed and disputed (see Case Example 59).

> **Case Example 59. Doubts about the decision**
>
> The following excerpt stems from therapy with a 76-year-old caregiving wife.
>
> *Caregiver:* Well, now, at the moment [slight laughter], where I'm hearing you again, I am not 100% convinced.
>
> *Therapist:* Okay, that changes too.
>
> *Caregiver:* Yes, yes, that changes too, yes.
>
> *Therapist:* Mm-hmm. What could give you strength in moments when you doubt? What could help you not falter again and again, which is also very exhausting.
>
> *Caregiver:* Hmm [sigh]. I don't know. I can just – it just comes over more, I can't control it. If, for example, he smiles at me like this or hugs me or something, and so ... oh ...
>
> *Therapist:* But that's not gone.
>
> *Caregiver:* Yes.
>
> *Therapist:* It's not gone. You can continue to have that when you visit him, when you do something with him. Then you can continue to cultivate your relationship.
>
> *Caregiver:* Yes, true.
>
> *Therapist:* And you can do good again.
>
> *Caregiver:* Yes, so for me that's ... that he can get out. When I saw how exhausting that was. And when I imagine that he just had to stay inside this space, limited by the kitchen, living room, bedroom, nothing more, bathroom – yes, that's not fulfilling either.
>
> *Therapist:* So, I – yes, what's so lovely when you're with your husband. No one can take that from you.
>
> *Caregiver:* Yes. Oh yes, that ... um. So, at the moment I have that feeling of relief again [slight laughter] that I think: "Oh yes, that's all good."
>
> *Therapist:* I think I asked you the question earlier, about what could help you if you have such serious doubts and this guilty conscience that you should nurse your husband until the end. I think it would be good if you do something to push against that. So, when you notice that you are under so much pressure inside – what can you say to yourself, what gives you strength again, what gives you clarity again, what ... yes, takes away the doubt a little.
>
> *Caregiver:* Mm-hmm.
>
> *Therapist:* Do you have any ideas on what could help you at the moment?

Caregiver: Yes, then, yes, then I think, then I think about rolling him into the café in his wheelchair, because then he'll eat some cake [laughs].

Therapist: Yes, yes, exactly. Perhaps to imagine it really as an image. Something lovely that is possible there that is not possible at home right now.

Caregiver: Yes, that's ... that's ... yes, he likes that too. He'll like that too. Cake is his passion and um ... Yes, then I can put him in his wheelchair and walk with him – or even in the pedestrian zone through the shops. So, that's what I'm really looking forward to now [laughs].

Therapist: Exactly, that's something really nice to imagine. He likes to look around, likes to be outside. The cars, the people, the shops. Then enjoy a piece of cake together and provide him quality of life. Yes. Try this inner image of what you have there, as you – I don't know [slight laughter] – are walking through the shopping mall with him, and maybe he is sitting in a wheelchair. Then really pull yourself up in such a moment and use your imagination, so you are not in doubt again and again – to provide yourself with certainty ... no, that's good and to look forward to it and to use it to push against the doubt.

Caregiver: Yes, that is a good idea. That ... yes, I hadn't really imagined that yet. But when I think about it now, he's having fun. Yes, well, that's a good idea. I will then imagine that. And when I imagine it that way now [slight laughter]: it's a shame that it hasn't come to that yet!

If family caregivers initially choose to continue the care at the end of the decision-making process, but then at a later point in time have the feeling that they can no longer guarantee care due to changes in the caregiving situation (e.g., a strong progression of the dementia syndrome), then a new decision-making process will be set in motion. Then again, the use of pros and cons checklists can be helpful (see Worksheet 13-1: Should I Utilize Support?).

It is also important to prepare the situation in which the person with dementia should be informed of the decision to place them in a home. Family caregivers are often unsure whether the person with dementia can understand and comprehend the situation or the motives and how they will react if the caregivers suggest nursing-home care. Helpful ideas are provided in Questions 24.

Questions 24. Clarifying ideas with the family caregivers

- How do I tell them?
- How do I explain to them that I can no longer provide care at home and that they would be better if they were cared for in a home?
- When is the best time to tell them? As late as possible so that they do not get so upset or as early as possible so that they can adjust to it?

14.4 Care in an Emergency

Often the person with dementia needs to be placed in a nursing home due to an acute emergency or an illness on short notice. A nursing home admission often follows after a hospital stay. Then there is usually little time for preparations. Since spontaneous admission suddenly leads to extensive life changes and the family caregivers are overwhelmed, it is important to accompany and support them in this process. As a preventative measure, the therapist can encourage family caregivers to take precautions for such situations. There are various preparations to be made for this:

- inspecting and selecting a facility in case of an emergency, e.g., a short-term care facility, or nursing home;
- if possible or necessary, registering in advance at the chosen facility;
- placing necessary documents, such as ID and telephone numbers, in an easily accessible place; and
- informing neighbors and family of the steps to be taken in an emergency.

Worksheet 13-2: Emergency Plan can be used. In Case Example 60, the caregiving daughter did not have time to take these precautions due to an acute emergency, which was very burdensome for her.

The case example shows that it makes sense to discuss the issue of the emergency situation with family caregivers at an early stage in the course of therapy. Further information and examples for the development of possi-

> **Case Example 60. Nursing home placement after hospitalization**
>
> The following excerpt stems from therapy with a 43-year-old caregiving daughter.
>
> *Therapist:* How did you deal with the fact that your father had to go to a nursing home so quickly?
>
> *Caregiver:* Um ... it was very difficult for me because it happened so quickly, and I was the one who had to take care of everything. So, I went with him to the hospital to have him put on medication, and then we had to look for a home from there. It all had to happen very quickly. And then, I picked him up at the hospital and brought him to the nursing home. My father told me at the home: "If you leave me here, I'll kill myself." That was horrible for me.
>
> *Therapist:* That was horrible. That hurt you very much.
>
> *Caregiver:* Yes. But I just couldn't do it any other way.
>
> *Therapist:* You couldn't, exactly.
>
> *Caregiver:* And I can still remember a situation where my father once implied that he just doesn't know everything anymore or doesn't know his way around anymore. And then I said: "Oh, it's best not to think about it." Now I think we should have talked to him at the time and taken precautions. But, as the child, you are full of inhibitions and don't really know where to start.
>
> *Therapist:* I think the impression that you should have talked earlier arises from today's knowledge. I would say that in the situation back then, you probably were not able to see in advance what would come to you and how you could prepare yourself.
>
> *Caregiver:* Yes, I think so too.

ble courses of action and their preparation in an emergency can be found in Chapter 13.

14.5 Dealing With the Decision

Since the nursing process by the family caregivers is not completed after the nursing-home placement but continues to be very stressful and painful for many caregivers, support should be offered to family caregivers even after their family member with dementia has entered the nursing home. The transition from care at home to a nursing home is a drastic experience for most family caregivers. The move to a nursing home should, therefore, be well prepared for the family member with dementia and for the caregivers. The full extent of the change usually becomes apparent to the family caregivers when the family member with dementia enters the home. The loss is then experienced as real and painful, as Case Example 61 illustrates.

The placement of a family member with dementia in a nursing home is often experienced as ambivalent and very painful: On the one hand, the stressful situation caused by caregiving is put into perspective; on the other hand, caregivers may have the feeling that they have failed in caregiving. In the literature, this is described as the "parallelism of relief and loss" (German: "Parallelität von Entlastung und Verlust"; Schmidt, 2005). The emotionally stressful situation when a family member suffering from dementia moves into a nursing home is also caused by the family caregivers' insecurity regarding whether they have made the right decision.

Therefore, family caregivers should be supported in their decision by validating the decision, since many family caregivers feel guilty and also struggle with accusations from their environment, for example from other family members. Here it is always important to emphasize the individual reasons for the admission to the nursing home and to support the family caregivers in their decision. This helps many caregivers to cope better with feelings of guilt.

In handing over the care that has defined the caregivers' lives for a long period of time, an emptiness arises for them that must be processed. The therapist can use methods from Chapter 12 to support processing. In addition, admission to a care home can result in major changes in the family's financial situation that need to be addressed (see Case Example 62).

Case Example 61. Grief after nursing-home placement

Caregiver: On Monday, we put my mother in a home.

Therapist: [Takes a deep breath], Ok, so, so fast, yes?

Caregiver: Yes. In fact, the events started happening so fast. After our session last week, the facility called: "There is a spot available *now*."

Therapist: Okay. So, that ... that happened a little too fast for you now.

Caregiver: Yes.

Therapist: Okay. That ... of course, I didn't expect that right now either, you know.

Caregiver: Yes.

Therapist: Last week, we made a pros and cons list. And now you say that you are doing badly.

Caregiver: Yes.

Therapist: Mm-hmm.

Caregiver: So ... of course, I miss her now. Um, there are of course, situations, for example, yesterday morning before I went to work: I had a lot of time, and I enjoyed that. Or when I came back from swimming on Monday. We took her away on Monday, and then I went swimming in the evening, and um ... afterwards I didn't have to get her ready for bed, ... so then I could also – although I didn't sleep at night either, I can hear her at night although she is no longer there.

Therapist: Okay. Well, now, at first, there's a ... probably an incredible void that your mother has left behind. So, she was always present ... and ...

Caregiver: Yes. And I go there every day. But when I'm there and see [crying] the empty room or her things sitting there or something like that ... it really affects me.

Therapist: So that you really miss her, right?

Caregiver: Yes.

Therapist: So, actually, that's also – how should I put it? – something very valuable, yes, that you also notice what your mother means to you. You can now feel it so intensely, how important she is to you, how close she is to you.

Case Example 62. Dealing with the decision for nursing-home placement

The following excerpt stems from therapy with an 83-year-old caregiving wife.

Caregiver: It's difficult when you always sit alone in the evening and ponder ... and sometimes the questions arise: "Was it right or was it not right? Could you have kept him at home?" But it ... it wouldn't have taken long, then I would have had a breakdown. That wouldn't have been possible.

Therapist: Yes, I think so too, and that was definitely the right decision. You have looked after and nursed your husband for a very long time. And anyone who knows your situation a little better can understand that now was simply the time to hand over the care. And you haven't made it easy for yourself in any way.

Caregiver: Yes. But sometimes, the guilty conscience comes. For example, yesterday I went to our bakery and bought a cake for us. The saleswoman asked me where my husband was. When I told her that he is now in the nursing home, she said in astonishment that he still looked so fit. Well, and then I get a strange feeling.

Therapist: I can understand that well. Many family caregivers experience such situations because the disease is often not so obvious to outsiders. You have to know the person with dementia very well and experience them frequently in everyday life in order to be able to judge how severely limited they are. You know that very well, however. Because you have looked after him around the clock every day of the week, pushing your own physical limits.

Caregiver: Yes, that's true. But it still makes me sad.

Therapist: Yes, I can understand that. That is also quite normal in this situation. You have been married for so long and always went to the bakery together. Who wouldn't be sad?

Caregiver: Yes, that's true. And I am very happy that my husband has settled in there so well, that he feels comfortable there. Because that's really been bothering me. I wouldn't have thought that at all. I've had bad dreams for the past few nights. Sometimes the thought occurs to me: Wouldn't it still have been possible to keep him here? But ... I know, it's ... everyone says: "What you did was right."

Therapist: Yes, it was right. Most certainly. And, as a result, not only has your husband's life changed, your life has also changed completely. And it will certainly take a while until you have settled into this new situation.

Caregiver: Yes, I think so, too.

Therapist: Perhaps we can recollect the reasons for the home placement that you listed back then and what you had planned for the time after the admission to the home.

Caregiver: Yes, it just didn't work at home anymore. My health wasn't good at all. And I immediately liked the home. I looked at all of them nearby. The room is nice, the nurses are very nice. And when it gets warmer again, I'll go for a walk in the park with my husband. And I'll go swimming again too. And I've already bought a laptop so that I can write down my memories for my grandchildren. But I haven't gotten to that yet.

Therapist: That's great!

A home admission can also create resources for the person with dementia, since the care tasks and housekeeping are taken over by nursing staff, thus providing relief for the family caregivers. Contact with the person with dementia can thus be more intensive again. This can be helpful for dealing with the loss.

In this phase, it can also be helpful to remind the family caregivers of their own pro arguments and to make them aware that the quality of the relationship with the family member with dementia has often not changed at all or has sometimes even improved. In Case Example 63, the differentiation between the quantity of care concerning the personal time and communication spent together is emphasized. This differentiation can help family caregivers not only in making decisions but also in particular with respect to dealing with and accepting the reality of nursing-home placement.

Case Example 63. Promoting acceptance of the decision

Therapist: And if you take a look for yourself, that is, to the time before, when your mother was still living in your home, the time you spent together was quantitatively a lot, so to speak, where you were close, spatial closeness. The amount of time together has, of course, shrunk considerably. The quantity of time has changed. But the quality time, how has that changed?

Caregiver: Yes, I hadn't seen it that way before, yes. Yes, we now go into town, and there are a lot of people, and she has a lot to look at, and then she gets her piece of cake.

Therapist: Lovely.

Caregiver: And that is a time that we completely have together – or if the weather is not so good, then I always bring her a piece of cake, which she eats there, sometimes in the fresh air on her balcony. And then she eats it. Then she no longer sees what's left and right when she has her cake.

Therapist: [laughs]

Caregiver: That's her highlight of the day.

Therapist: I think that is something very valuable, what you have together and what you enable your mother to do. That you spend so much time with her is valuable. Very valuable time.

Caregiver: Yes, that's, that's right. Yes, I have never seen it in such a way that these 1 or 2 hours that we are together in the city are very intense. Yes, that is true. I didn't have that much time with her before. Always only in between. When we drank coffee, I would sit there with her, then I also drank coffee.

Therapist: Yes, what do you take with you from the conversation today?

Caregiver: Um, yes, above all, that you have now made me aware of how intensively I experience this free time with my mother. These are all things that I wasn't really aware of. So, that I always had her around me here, but I still didn't do anything with her, so intensively. That I've realized this now is good. Now that my mother is in a nursing home, I can ultimately do a lot more with her than at home because she is being nursed anyway.

Therapist: Exactly. Hmm ... keep that understanding, will you? Make yourself aware every now and then. In times when you feel so doubtful that you make it clear to yourself again.

Caregiver: Yes.

14.6 Therapeutic Procedure for Intolerable Caregiving Situations

An intolerable caregiving situation is illustrated in Case Example 64.

If a situation of violence in caregiving becomes apparent, this often means that the therapist is faced with an internal stress test in terms of maintaining the relationship with the caregiver and making decisions to protect the person with dementia.

Families often avoid addressing violence, local contact persons are unknown, and doctors and nurses sometimes avoid open discussion. These circumstances make it considerably more difficult for the therapist to take necessary steps and action. Possible therapeutic approaches for such situations are now presented (see also Bonillo et al., 2013).

If it becomes clear that the person with dementia is being violently attacked, then first clarify:
- What exactly does the violence look like?
- Are there any doubts regarding the violence reported by the caregiver? (What speaks for it, what speaks against it?)

First, strategies for emotion regulation (see Chapters 9 and 10) should be discussed with the caregiver, and their implementation in daily life should be specifically and repeatedly asked about. If it becomes apparent that the violence persists, is believable, there is no motivation to change from the caregiver, and there is no reduction in the occurrence of violent attacks, then the therapist should initiate measures to protect the person with dementia. Ideally, the family caregiver will be willing to organize support and change the situation themselves before the therapist feels obliged to take any action. If the family caregiver decide against a change and against taking action themselves, the therapist must adhere to the regulations on confidentiality.

Laws on confidentiality, on which information is protected under confidentiality, and on breaching confidentiality vary from country to country and from jurisdiction to jurisdiction. It is, therefore, imperative for the therapist to inform themselves about laws on confidentiality in the jurisdiction in which therapy is practiced.

Maintaining confidentiality is a very valuable asset and must not be broken. This means that the therapist must not breach confidentiality! However, after careful consideration, and in accordance with respective criminal laws, confidentiality can be broken, and necessary steps can be taken if a person's life or health is acutely and immediately endangered, and disclosure can prevent further damage. On an individual basis, it should be considered very carefully which aspect outweighs the other: protection of privacy for the family caregiver or protection against possible danger for the person with dementia.

> **Case Example 64. Intolerable caregiving situation: Violence against the person with dementia**
>
> The following excerpt stems from therapy with a 56-year-old caregiving daughter.
>
> *Caregiver:* Yesterday I burst with anger again. She soiled the house again. The diaper was on the floor and the smell was everywhere in the house … *disgusting!* So, I went to her, and I grabbed her arm and said to her, "Don't do that again, I've had enough with you." Then she just says that she'll tell my brother. Well, he should come by, he never shows up here. She provokes me too! So, it was the last straw for me.
>
> *Therapist:* How did the situation continue?
>
> *Caregiver:* I said, "Get in your bed now." Well again, she didn't want to. Well, now she has bruises. She always gets them right away.
>
> *Therapist:* What do you mean, she's got bruises now, from what? You said you grabbed her arm.
>
> *Caregiver:* Yes, I had had enough. I was boiling. And when she didn't go to bed, well … I helped her. Yes, I know you don't like that, but what else am I supposed to do? She's as stubborn as a goat.
>
> *Therapist:* Yes, I really don't like that. You already told me last time that sometimes your hand slips too.
>
> *Caregiver:* I don't put up with it anymore – she has to learn somehow that the diaper has to stay on.
>
> *Therapist:* Have there been other situations where you've been rough with her, and it wasn't about the diaper?
>
> *Caregiver:* Well, when she resists washing. But I have to: I won't leave her lying in her own feces and then put up with the stench. That's where I reach my limit.
>
> *Therapist:* In the last session, we talked about strategies for dealing with your anger. We also already talked about incontinence and thought about how you can deal with it better. Did you try anything out?
>
> *Caregiver:* No, I did not. When would I have time to? I'm taking care of everything here by myself.
>
> *Therapist:* That really worries me, Ms. A. I don't think this situation is tolerable. This is not how things should be done.
>
> *Caregiver:* Mm-hmm.
>
> *Therapist:* We had already talked about the possibility of placing your mother in a home.
>
> *Caregiver:* I have already told you that that's not possible. That just won't work, financially and everything. We don't want to give up our property here and everything.
>
> *Therapist:* But it also doesn't work when you get into situations where you lose control. I come into a conflict here and can no longer support you if you are not willing to change something about it.
>
> *Caregiver:* Well, what do you want to do now?

While carefully assessing the individual situation, these questions should be considered:
- What consequences would a report have for the family caregivers? (*criminal*: possibly financial and/or probation; *psychosocial*: e.g., increase in conflict in the family, withdrawal from their social environment; *mental*: negative consequences for their self-image, damage of trust in professional help)
- What are the consequences of a report for the person with dementia? (possibly no change in the caregiving situation, then danger for increasing escalation; change in the caregiving situation)
- For the therapist: What are the consequences of a report/notification to the mental health court for the therapist? (possibly having to testify as a witness, actively oppose the client, hurt the therapeutic relationship massively, and live with the negative consequences for the family caregivers, their social environment, and for the person living with dementia)

Regardless of what the therapist decides to do, it is particularly important to document the therapy sessions precisely and to have contact with lawyers and local authorities to clarify possible help and legal issues. It is also essential for the therapist to document their own reflection during the process of considering whether to initiate taking action.

One initial approach could be that the therapist contacts the district in which the caregiver resides to find out who the local contacts are for violence in caregiving. This alone can be time consuming, involving several telephone calls to find the person responsible. For example, in larger cities, the city's senior citizens' representation can provide information about local contact points (care authority, social-psychiatric services, possibly geriatric-psychiatric services, and public health officers). Insurance companies can also provide information on nursing advisors who can offer support and, if available, home visits. In rural areas, the infrastructure in this regard can be unclear and insufficient. Therefore, it can be difficult in some regions to find out where possible responsible persons are located. The social-psychiatric service is often the place to contact and can send someone to make home visits.

Once the therapist has inquired about the persons responsible and possibilities, the family caregivers should be given the opportunity to inform the contact person, for example the caregiving advisor or the social-psychiatric service, themselves, and to organize receiving help and support. Therefore, the therapist should initially

> **Case Example 65. Intolerable caregiving situation: Violence against the person with dementia (continuation of Case Example 64)**
>
> *Therapist:* Ms. A., in our last session you promised me that you would get help regarding the situation with your mother. You wanted to contact a caregiving advisor at your insurance company and you wanted to, above all, address that you are having problems in dealing with your mother.
>
> *Caregiver:* Yes, I did that. It took a lot of effort for me, but I called them.
>
> *Therapist:* Brilliant! I think that's really good. How did the conversation go?
>
> *Caregiver:* Well, we made an appointment for Ms. Z. to come here, she would like to see the situation for herself.
>
> *Therapist:* I'm happy about that, great! How are you doing with it?
>
> *Caregiver:* Yes, I am relieved, I think. She was very nice.
>
> *Therapist:* Yes. That's good. And she's coming over?
>
> *Caregiver:* Yes, next week, on the 8th.
>
> *Therapist:* Okay. Would it be okay with you if I checked with Ms. Z. that you have informed her? Don't get me wrong, I trust you, but I just want to make sure.
>
> *Caregiver:* Yes, yes, I understand. I already told her that you can call.
>
> *Therapist:* Ok, thank you. Then I will do that.
>
> *Caregiver:* I also talked to my sister.
>
> *Therapist:* Yes, great!
>
> *Caregiver:* And she thinks that we should put our mother in a home.
>
> *Therapist:* Yes, what do you think about that?
>
> *Caregiver:* Well, I don't know how it's supposed to work financially. I have to think about it. It was always my goal to keep the house here. But I have understood now that I can't do that at all costs.
>
> *Therapist:* Yes, you have realized that now?
>
> *Caregiver:* Yes.
>
> *Therapist:* Yes, a lot has been going on lately.
>
> *Caregiver:* Yes, somehow. I first have to talk to Ms. Z. and find out about the finances and such, but I'm already playing with the idea.
>
> *Therapist:* Okay, that sounds good. You're dealing with it.
>
> *Caregiver:* Yes, I've started to.

inquire anonymously. Suppose the family caregiver is not willing to get support, which could be associated with negative financial consequences (e.g., loss of nursing allowances). After weighing the factors mentioned, the therapist can find a contact person responsible in the local district to contact and visit the family. The family caregiver should be informed about the contact.

Such a decision can lead to the termination of the therapeutic relationship. However, "playing through" possible consequences (the therapist talks about possibly reporting the problem) can lead to the family caregiver adopting a clear motivation for change and thus taking the initiative and organizing support to correct their own problematic behavior and/or ending home care and placing their family member in a nursing home. Case Example 65 continues with the intolerable caregiving situation raised in Case Example 64.

Information on the subject of violence in caregiving with helpful recommendations for action and information on legal aspects can be found in the review by Harrigan (2010) or in the book "Safeguarding People With Dementia" from the Alzheimer's Society UK (n.d.).

15 Completion of Therapy

The completion of therapy with family caregivers should be prepared in the long term. Due to the caregiving situation, a large number of family caregivers are socially isolated and the therapy sometimes represents the most important or an important form of social contact. The challenge for therapists is to find an appropriate closure of the therapy while at the same time knowing that the illness of the person with dementia will continue to worsen and that there may still be many challenges ahead for the family caregivers.

15.1 Goals of the Module

The final phase focuses primarily on summarizing the goals achieved, collecting coping options developed in therapy, and ensuring that the changes and successes achieved are maintained. Moreover, family caregivers should be prepared for upcoming crises (further deterioration of dementia, death of the family member with dementia). Furthermore, therapists can discuss with caregivers which additional support offers they can seek out and utilize in order to receive long-term support. Obtaining feedback and saying goodbye is also important. Box 23 contains an overview of the interventions covered in this chapter.

Box 23. Overview of the interventions

- Evaluating the achieved goals
- Gathering coping options and maintaining achieved changes
- Dealing with crises
- Utilization of further support options
- Feedback to the therapist
- Saying goodbye

15.2 Therapeutic Approach

15.2.1 Evaluating the Achieved Goals

Using Goal Attainment Scaling (Kiresuk & Sherman, 1968) from the initial interview (see Worksheet 7-2: Checklist for Defining a Target State), progress and successes achieved in therapy can be discussed with the family caregivers. Questions 25 are therefore helpful.

Questions 25. Discussing the achieved goals

- For each goal: To which extent did you reach your goal?
- How far have you come toward your goals?
- What is still missing?
- Where is there still something to be done or where is there still potential for further development?

Even each small change should be positively reinforced and recorded in writing. In addition, an assessment should be made on the Goal Attainment Scaling with respect to what extent the goals discussed at the beginning of therapy could be achieved, from +3 (extreme improvement) to −1 (deterioration).

It can also be discussed with the family caregivers which goals they would like to continue working on in the future and what this might entail in concrete terms. For example, a family caregiver who formulated the goal in the first session of wanting to pursue more pleasant activities in the future, in the form of swimming once a week and meeting with a friend, realizes in the final session that she could only achieve this goal partially. She only managed to comply with these wishes once a month. At this point, existing hurdles and ways to pursue the goal in the future can be discussed once again.

Some family caregivers may also find that the goals set at the beginning of therapy no longer correspond to their needs and, for example, were more like socially desirable goals. In such cases, it can be useful to work out again what the main needs of the caregivers are and how these can be met. It should be recorded again in writing which goals have been achieved, which are to be worked on further, and/or which are to be maintained so that there will be no deterioration in the caregiver's condition.

15.2.2 Gathering Coping Options and Maintaining Achieved Changes

In the final phase of therapy, it is reasonable to summarize the acquired coping options so that they can be further implemented and maintained in the caregivers' everyday life in the long term. Here, as shown in Box 24, the use of metaphors can be helpful.

Box 24. Metaphor for learning new behaviors

> "Imagine you were on vacation and started riding a horse (or painting, or something similar). You practiced there with a riding instructor and were quite successful in saddling the horse, mounting it, moving to different gaits, and finally riding it through the landscape. You really enjoyed it and noticed how good it made you feel. By now, you've been back from the trip for 4 months and haven't ridden again since then. How about your riding skills? What should be done? What would you recommend to someone who had such an experience on vacation and now comes back home? How can this be transferred to therapy? How could you retain and expand progress?"

Lists and plans can be drawn up with the caregivers, that, if necessary, can promote and ensure a continuation of what has been learned in therapy. The positively tried and tested strategies for coping with difficult situations can be written down on colorful flashcards, for example, that can be hung up in their home in clearly visible places. Depending on the caregivers' needs and life situation, these cards can contain, for example, taking regular breaks, consulting with a friend, treating themselves to something, utilizing short-term care.

15.2.3 Dealing With Crises

The course of dementia can cause family caregivers to be exposed again and again to new situations and crises. Since the end of psychotherapeutic support seldom coincides with the end of caregiving, it must be assumed that the family caregivers will have to deal with a multitude of new and stressful situations in the future as well. Even if the further course of the dementia cannot be foreseen, some precautions can be taken. Important information on the topic of admission to a nursing home and dealing with emergencies can be found, for example, in Chapter 14. It is wise to draw up emergency plans that can be used again at the end of therapy to check to which extent they are still valid or need to be changed (see Chapter 13).

The important topic of preparing for the death of the person with dementia can be addressed again in the final process. Information on this can be found in Chapter 12. Helpful explanations concerning the time before and after the death of the person with dementia (such as grief is normal, plans for the time after the sick person's death) can be recalled and written down. In addition, signals can also be collected that could, for example, indicate the caregiver's feeling of being overburdened. A list of "warning signs" for overburdening (e.g., severe physical exhaustion, sleep disorders, brooding, lack of drive), similar to relapse prevention for depression, can be made.

15.2.4 Utilization of Additional Support Services

In the final phase, the transition to a self-help group can be discussed and prepared with the family caregivers. In addition, family caregivers should be given contact information for local support organizations (for example, offers from the Alzheimer's association). Questions regarding dementia symptoms, diagnosis, dealing with problem behaviors, legal questions, self-help groups, or other individual caregiving problems can be asked here.

Moreover, all professional support options collected during the therapy should be listed again so that the family caregivers are prepared for future situations in which the utilization of additional professional support is required.

15.2.5 Feedback to the Therapist

Therapists should also use the opportunity to obtain feedback on their work and therapy. Therapists should emphasize that it is particularly important to receive suggestions for improvement in order to be able to develop further.

Questions 26 provides an overview of some sample questions that the therapists can ask the family caregivers.

Questions 26. Obtaining feedback

> - Overall, how satisfied are you with the outcome of the therapy?
> - Which aspects of the psychological support did you find especially helpful? What did you like?
> - Which aspects of the psychological support bothered you and which, in your opinion, could be improved?
> - Which important topics were you able to address during the psychological support?
> - Was something missing?
> - How did the psychological support help you to deal with your problems more appropriately?
> - How could you transfer what you learned in therapy to your everyday life?

The experience has shown that most family caregivers perceive psychological support to be very helpful and relieving. Individual feedback from family caregivers for the therapy is shown in the following Examples.

Examples. Feedback from family caregivers

> "My point of view and way of thinking has changed a lot! Through the talks with you I was also able to improve my behavior toward my family member with dementia, but also toward other people in a positive way! I have become more self-confident and calmer. ..."

> Although I still continue to feel desperate at times, I am able to straighten myself out again and say to myself: You are capable of lovingly caring for your family member and living through the difficult years with him! At the same time, I am able to arrange time for myself too!"

> "I feel better now, I have become more confident in dealing with the disease, have opened myself up to new possibilities, things have become a lot easier, and my fears have declined."

> "When I applied for Tele.TAnDem I thought that I couldn't really be taught anything anymore. I thought that I already had caregiving under complete control. That I learned during the sessions to care about myself and to also take care of myself – without neglecting caregiving – has been a huge benefit!"

15.2.6 Saying Goodbye

Finally, it is important to use personal and positive-regard-related words and to express best wishes to the caregivers for the continuing caregiving situation and the future. Depending on the previous course of therapy, booster sessions can be arranged or therapists can inform the caregivers that they can get in touch again in the event of a crisis. This, however, depends very much on the respective setting and formalities.

References

Alzheimer's Association. (2022). *About.* https://www.alz.org/about

Alzheimer's Society UK. (n.d.). *Safeguarding people with dementia.* https://shop.alzheimers.org.uk/helpful-products/books/safeguarding-people-with-dementia

Alzheimer's Society UK. (2018). *Selecting and moving into a care home.* https://www.alzheimers.org.uk/sites/default/files/2018-12/Alzheimers-Society_Selecting-and-Moving-in-to-a-New-Care-Home_181207.pdf

Alzheimer's Society UK. (2022). *Caring for a person with dementia: A practical guide.* https://www.alzheimers.org.uk/get-support/publications-factsheets/caring-person-dementia-practical-guide

American Psychiatric Association. (2013). *Diagnostic and statistical manual of mental disorders* (5th ed.). APA.

Annerstedt, L., Elmståhl, S., Ingvad, B., & Samuelsson, S. M. (2000). Family caregiving in dementia: An analysis of the caregiver's burden and the "breaking-point" when home care becomes inadequate. *Scandinavian Journal of Public Health, 28*(1), 23-31.

Atienza, A. A., Collins, R., & King, A. C. (2001). The mediating effects of situational control on social support and mood following a stressor: A prospective study of dementia caregivers in their natural environments. Journals of Gerontology. *Series B, Psychological Sciences and Social Sciences, 56*(3), 129-139. https://doi.org/10.1093/geronb/56.3.S129

Bambach, S. (2006). *5-4-3-2-1-Methode* [5-4-3-2-1 Method]. In O. Schubbe (Ed.), *Traumatherapie mit EMDR. Ein Handbuch für die Ausbildung* [Trauma therapy using EMDR. A manual for education] (pp. 248-253). Vandenhoeck & Ruprecht.

Barrera-Caballero, S., Romero-Moreno, R., Pedroso-Chaparro, M. D., Olmos, R., Vara-García, C., Gallego-Alberto, L., Cabrera, I., Márquez-González, M., Olazarán, J., & Losada-Baltar, A. (2021). Stress, cognitive fusion and comorbid depressive and anxiety symptomatology in dementia caregivers. *Psychology and Aging, 36*(5), 667-676.

Beach, S. R., Schulz, R., Williamson, G. M., Miller, L. S., Weiner, M. F., & Lance, C. E. (2005). Risk factors for potentially harmful informal caregiver behavior. *Journal of the American Geriatrics Society, 53*(2), 255-261. https://doi.org/10.1111/j.1532-5415.2005.53111.x

Belle, S. H., Burgio, L., Burns, R., Coon, D., Czaja, S. J., Gallagher-Thompson, D., Gitlin, L. N., Klinger, J., Koepke, K. M., Lee, C. C., Martindale-Adam, J., Nichols, L., Schulz, R., Stahl, S., Stevens, A., Winter, L., & Zhang, S. (2006). Enhancing the quality of life of dementia caregivers from different ethnic or racial groups: A randomized, controlled trial. *Annals of Internal Medicine, 145*(10), 727-738.

Bieber, A., Nguyen, N., Meyer, G., & Stephan, A. (2019). Influences on the access to and use of formal community care by people with dementia and their informal caregivers: A scoping review. *BMC Health Services Research, 19*(1), 88. https://doi.org/10.1186/s12913-018-3825-z

Bjørge, H., Sæteren, B., & Ulstein, I. D. (2019). Experience of companionship among family caregivers of persons with dementia: A qualitative study. *Dementia: International Journal of Social Research and Practice, 18*(1), 228-244. https://doi.org/10.1177/1471301216666172

Boerner, K., Schulz, R., & Horowitz, A. (2004). Positive aspects of caregiving and adaptation to bereavement. *Psychology and Aging, 19*(4), 668-675. https://doi.org/10.1037/0882-7974.19.4.668

Bonillo, M., Heidenblut, S., Philipp-Metzen, E., Saxl, S., Schacke, C., Steinhusen, C., Wilhelm, I., & Zank, S. (2013). *Gewalt in der familialen Pflege: Prävention, Früherkennung, Intervention – Ein Manual für die ambulante Pflege* [Violence in family care: Prevention, early recognition, intervention – A manual for outpatient care]. Kohlhammer. https://doi.org/10.17433/978-3-17-024026-1

Bowlby, J. (1977). The making and breaking of affectional bonds. I. Aetiology and psychopathology in the light of attachment theory. An expanded version of the Fifth Maudsley Lecture, delivered before the Royal College of Psychiatrists, 19 November 1976. *British Journal of Psychiatry: The Journal of Mental Science, 130*, 201-210.

Bressan, V., Visintini, C., & Palese, A. (2020). What do family caregivers of people with dementia need? A mixed-method systematic review. *Health & Social Care in the Community, 28*(6), 1942-1960. https://doi.org/10.1111/hsc.13048

Brodaty, H., Thomson, C., Thompson, C., & Fine, M. (2005). Why caregivers of people with dementia and memory loss don't use services. *International Journal of Geriatric Psychiatry, 20*(6), 537-546. https://doi.org/10.1002/gps.1322

Cabote, C. J., Bramble, M., & McCann, D. (2015). Family caregivers' experiences of caring for a relative with younger onset dementia: A qualitative systematic review. *Journal of Family Nursing, 21*(3), 443–468. https://doi.org/10.1177/1074840715573870

Cheng, S. T. (2017). Dementia caregiver burden: A research update and critical analysis. *Current Psychiatry Reports, 19*(9), 64. https://doi.org/10.1007/s11920-017-0818-2

Cheng, S. T., Au, A., Losada, A., Thompson, L. W., & Gallagher-Thompson, D. (2019). Psychological interventions for dementia caregivers: What we have achieved, what we have learned. *Current Psychiatry Reports, 21*(7), 59. https://doi.org/10.1007/s11920-019-1045-9

Cheung, D. S. K., Ho, K. H. M., Cheung, T. F., Lam, S. C., & Tse, M. M. Y. (2018). Anticipatory grief of spousal and adult children caregivers of people with dementia. *BMC Palliative Care, 17*(1), 124. https://doi.org/10.1186/s12904-018-0376-3

Clark, S., Prescott, T., & Murphy, G. (2019). The lived experiences of dementia in married couple relationships. *Dementia: International Journal of Social Research and Practice, 18*(5), 1727–1739. https://doi.org/10.1177/1471301217722034

Coe, M., & Neufeld, A. (1999). Male caregivers' use of formal services. *Western Journal of Nursing Research, 21*, 568–588. https://doi.org/10.1177/01939459922044045

Coen, R. F., O'Boyle, C. A., Coakley, D., & Lawlor, B. A. (2002). Individual quality of life factors distinguishing low-burden and high-burden caregivers of dementia patients. *Dementia and Geriatric Cognitive Disorders, 13*(3), 164–170. https://doi.org/10.1159/000048648

Cohen, G., Russo, M. J., Campos, J. A., & Allegri, R. F. (2020). Living with dementia: Increased level of caregiver stress in times of COVID-19. *International Psychogeriatrics, 32*(11), 1377–1381. https://doi.org/10.1017/S1041610220001593

Collins, R. N., & Kishita, N. (2020). Prevalence of depression and burden among informal care-givers of people with dementia: A meta-analysis. *Ageing & Society, 40*(11), 2355–2392. https://doi.org/10.1017/S0144686X19000527

Coon, D. W., Thompson, L., Steffen, A., Sorocco, K., & Gallagher-Thompson, D. (2003). Anger and depression management: Psychoeducational skill training interventions for women caregivers of a relative with dementia. *The Gerontologist, 43*(5), 678–689. https://doi.org/10.1093/geront/43.5.678

Dehpour, T., & Koffman, J. (2023). Assessment of anticipatory grief in informal caregivers of dependants with dementia: A systematic review. *Aging & Mental Health, 27*(1), 110–123. https://doi.org/10.1080/13607863.2022.2032599

Dempsey, M., & Baago, S. (1998). Latent grief: The unique and hidden grief of carers of loved ones with dementia. *American Journal of Alzheimer's Disease and Other Dementias, 13*(2), 84–91. https://doi.org/10.1177/153331759801300206

Deutsche Alzheimer Gesellschaft e.V. Selbsthilfe Demenz. (2012a). *Inkontinenz in der häuslichen Versorgung Demenzkranker. Informationen und Tipps bei Blasen- und Darmschwäche* [Incontinence in home care for dementia patients: Information and tips for bladder and bowel weakness] (3rd ed., Vol. 8). Praxisreihe der Deutschen Alzheimer Gesellschaft e.V. Selbsthilfe Demenz.

Deutsche Alzheimer Gesellschaft e.V. Selbsthilfe Demenz. (2012b). *Leben mit Demenzkranken. Hilfen für schwierige Verhaltensweisen und Situationen im Alltag* [Living with dementia patients: Help for difficult behaviors and situations in everyday life] (6th ed., Vol. 5). Praxisreihe der Deutschen Alzheimer Gesellschaft e.V. Selbsthilfe Demenz.

Deutsche Alzheimer Gesellschaft e.V. Selbsthilfe Demenz. (2019). *Umzug ins Pflegeheim – Entscheidungshilfen für Angehörige von Menschen mit Demenz* [Moving to a nursing home: Decision-making aids for relatives of people with dementia] (3rd ed.). Praxisreihe der Deutschen Alzheimer Gesellschaft e.V. Selbsthilfe Demenz.

D'Zurilla, T. J., & Goldfried, M. R. (1971). Problem solving and behavior modification. *Journal of Abnormal Psychology, 78*(1), 107–126. https://doi.org/10.1037/h0031360

Eifert, G. H. (2011). *Akzeptanz- und Commitment-Therapie (ACT)* [Acceptance and commitment therapy (ACT)]. Hogrefe.

Eisdorfer, C., Czaja, S. J., Loewenstein, D. A., Rubert, M. P., Arguelles, S., Mitrani, V. B., & Szapocznik, J. (2003). The effect of a family therapy and technology-based intervention on caregiver depression. *The Gerontologist, 43*(4), 521–531. https://doi.org/10.1093/geront/43.4.521

Ellis, A. (1977). *Handbook of rational-emotive therapy*. Springer.

Enright, J., O'Connell, M. E., Branger, C., Kirk, A., & Morgan, D. (2020). Identity, relationship quality, and subjective burden in caregivers of persons with dementia. *Dementia: International Journal of Social Research and Practice, 19*(6), 1855–1871. https://doi.org/10.1177/1471301218808607

Eska, K., Graessel, E., Donath, C., Schwarzkopf, L., Lauterberg, J., & Holle, R. (2013). Predictors of institutionalization of dementia patients in mild and moderate stages: A 4-year prospective analysis. *Dementia and Geriatric Cognitive Disorders Extra, 3*(1), 426–445. https://doi.org/10.1159/000355079

Evans, R. L., & Baldwin, D. (1989). Factors affecting decision to participate in caregiver support groups. *Archives of Physical Medicine and Rehabilitation, 70*, 89.

Faschingbauer, T. R., Zisook, S., & DeVaul, R. (1987). The Texas Revised Inventory of Grief. In S. Zisook (Ed.), *Biopsychosocial aspects of bereavement* (pp. 109–124). American Psychiatric Press.

Fauth, E. B., & Gibbons, A. (2014). Which behavioral and psychological symptoms of dementia are the most problematic? Variability by prevalence, intensity, distress ratings, and associations with caregiver depressive symptoms. *International Journal of Geriatric Psychiatry, 29*(3), 263–271. https://doi.org/10.1002/gps.4002

Feil, N. (2012). *The validation breakthrough: Simple techniques for communicating with people with Alzheimer's and other dementias* (3rd ed.). Health Professions Press.

Feil, N., & de Klerk-Rubin, V. (2015). *V/F validation: The Feil method. How to help disoriented old-old* (3rd ed.). Edward Feil Productions.

Frank, J. B. (2008). Evidence for grief as the major barrier faced by Alzheimer caregivers: A qualitative analysis. *American Journal of Alzheimer's Disease & Other Dementias, 22*(6), 516–527. https://doi.org/10.1177/1533317507307787

Gage, M. J., & Kinney, J. M. (1995). They aren't for everyone: The impact of support group participation on caregiver's well-being. *Clinical Gerontologist, 16*, 21–34. https://doi.org/10.1300/J018v16n02_03

Gallagher-Thompson, D., Cassidy, E. L., & Lovett, S. (2000). Training psychologists for service delivery in long-term care settings. *Clinical Psychology: Science and Practice, 7*(3), 329–336. https://doi.org/10.1093/clipsy.7.3.329

Gallagher-Thompson, D., & Coon, D. W. (2007). Evidence-based psychological treatments for distress in family caregivers of older adults. *Psychology and Aging, 22*(1), 37–51. https://doi.org/10.1037/0882-7974.22.1.37

Gallagher-Thompson, D., Coon, D. W., Solano, N., Ambler, C., Rabinowitz, Y., & Thompson, L. W. (2003). Change in indices of distress among Latino and Anglo female caregivers of elderly relatives with dementia: Site-specific results from the REACH national collaborative study. *The Gerontologist, 43*(4), 580–591. https://doi.org/10.1093/geront/43.4.580

Gallagher-Thompson, D., Gray, H. L., Dupart, T., Jimenez, D., & Thompson, L. W. (2008). Effectiveness of cognitive/behavioral small group intervention for reduction of depression and stress in non-Hispanic white and Hispanic/Latino women dementia family caregivers: Outcomes and mediators of change. *Journal of Rational-Emotive & Cognitive-Behavior Therapy, 26*(4), 286–303. https://doi.org/10.1007/s10942-008-0087-4

GBD 2019 Dementia Forecasting Collaborators. (2022). Estimation of the global prevalence of dementia in 2019 and forecasted prevalence in 2050: An analysis for the Global Burden of Disease Study 2019. *Lancet Public Health, 7*(2), e105–e125. https://doi.org/10.1016/S2468-2667(21)00249-8

Geister, C. (2004). *"Weil ich für meine Mutter verantwortlich bin": Der Übergang von der Tochter zur pflegenden Tochter* ["Because I am responsible for my mother": The transition from a daughter to a caring daughter]. Hans Huber.

Gilhooly, K. J., Gilhooly, M. L. M., Sullivan, M. P., McIntyre, A., Wilson, L., Harding, E., Woodbridge, R., & Crutch, S. (2016). A meta-review of stress, coping and interventions in dementia and dementia caregiving. *BMC Geriatrics, 16*(106). https://doi.org/10.1186/s12877-016-0280-8

Glueckauf, R. L., Davis, W. S., Willis, F., Sharma, D., Gustafson, D. J., Hayes, J., Stutzman, M., Proctor, J., Kazmer, M. M., Murray, L., Shipman, J., McIntyre, V., Wesley, L., Schettini, G., Xu, J., Parfitt, F., Graff-Radford, N., Baxter, C., Burnett, K., ... Springer, J. (2012). Telephone-based, cognitive-behavioral therapy for African American dementia caregivers with depression: Initial findings. *Rehabilitation Psychology, 57*(2), 124–139.

Gouin, J. P., Hantsoo, L., & Kiecolt-Glaser, J. K. (2008). Immune dysregulation and chronic stress among older adults: A review. *Neuroimmunomodulation, 15*(4-6), 251–259. https://doi.org/10.1159/000156468

Grässel, E., Luttenberger, K., Römer, H., & Donath, C. (2010). Voluntary help in dementia: Predictors for utilisation and expected quality from a family caregiver's point of view. *Fortschritte der Neurologie-Psychiatrie, 78*(9), 536–541.

Hähnel, F. S., Töpfer, N. F., & Wilz, G. (2023). Effects of nursing home placement on the mental health trajectories of family caregivers of people with dementia: Findings from the Tele.TAnDem intervention study. *Aging & Mental Health, 27*(1), 101–109. https://doi.org/10.1080/13607863.2021.2022598

Halek, M., & Bartholomeyczik, S. (2006). *Verstehen und Handeln. Forschungsergebnisse zur Pflege von Menschen mit Demenz und herausforderndem Verhalten* [Understanding and acting: Research findings on caring for people with dementia and challenging behaviour]. Vandenhoeck & Ruprecht.

Harrigan, M. (2010). *Older adult abuse and dementia: A literature review*. Alzheimer Society of Canada. https://alzheimer.ca/sites/default/files/documents/Older-adult-abuse-and-dementia_Alzheimer-Society-Canada.pdf

Haupt, M. (1999). Der Verlauf von Verhaltensstörungen und ihre psychosoziale Behandlung bei Demenzkranken [The course of behavioural disorders and their psychosocial treatment in patients with dementia]. *Zeitschrift für Gerontologie und Geriatrie, 32*, 159–166. https://doi.org/10.1007/s003910050100

Haupt, M., Kurz, A., & Janner, M. (2000). A 2-year follow-up of behavioural and psychological symptoms in Alzheimer's disease. *Dementia and Geriatric Cognitive Disorders, 11*(3), 147–152. https://doi.org/10.1159/000017228

Hautzinger, M. (2000). *Depression im Alter (Materialien für die klinische Praxis)* [Depression in old age (materials for clinical practice)]. Beltz Psychologie Verlags Union (PVU).

Hebert, R. S., Dang, Q. Y., & Schulz, R. (2006). Preparedness for the death of a loved one and mental health in bereaved caregivers of patients with dementia: Findings from the REACH study. *Journal of Palliative Medicine, 9*(3), 683–693. https://doi.org/10.1089/jpm.2006.9.683

Hebert, R. S., & Schulz, R. (2006). Caregiving at the end of life. *Journal of Palliative Medicine, 9*(5), 1174–1187. https://doi.org/10.1089/jpm.2006.9.1174

Hedtke-Becker, A. (1990). *Die Pflegenden pflegen: Gruppen für Angehörige pflegebedürftiger alter Menschen: Eine Arbeitshilfe.* [Caring for carers: Groups for relatives of elderly people in need of care: A working guide]. Lambertus.

Holley, C. K., & Mast, B. T. (2009). The impact of anticipatory grief on caregiver burden in dementia caregivers. *The Gerontologist, 49*(3), 388–396. https://doi.org/10.1093/geront/gnp061

Holst, G., & Edberg, A. K. (2011). Wellbeing among people with dementia and their next of kin over a period of 3 years. *Scandinavian Journal of Caring Sciences, 25*(3), 549–557. https://doi.org/10.1111/j.1471-6712.2010.00863.x

Hooker, K., Bowman, S. R., Coehlo, D. P., Lim, S. R., Kaye, J., Guariglia, R., & Li, F. Z. (2002). Behavioral change in persons with dementia: Relationships with mental and physical health of caregivers. *Journals of Gerontology Series B: Psychological Sciences and Social Sciences, 57*(5), 453–460. https://doi.org/10.1093/geronb/57.5.P453

Hopkinson, M. D., Reavell, J., Lane, D. A., & Mallikarjun, P. (2019). Cognitive behavioral therapy for depression, anxiety, and stress in caregivers of dementia patients: A systematic review and meta-analysis. *The Gerontologist, 59*(4), 343–362. https://doi.org/10.1093/geront/gnx217

Höwler, E. (2008). *Herausforderndes Verhalten bei Menschen mit Demenz: Erleben und Strategien Pflegender* [Challenging behaviour in people with dementia: Carers' experiences and strategies]. Kohlhammer.

Huang, S. S. (2022). Depression among caregivers of patients with dementia: Associative factors and management approaches. *World Journal of Psychiatry, 12*(1), 59–76. https://doi.org/10.5498/wjp.v12.i1.59

Hurt, C., Bhattacharyya, S., Burns, A., Camus, V., Liperoti, R., Marriott, A., Nobili, F., Robert, P., Tsolaki, M., Vellas, B., Verhey, F., & Byrne, E. J. (2008). Patient and caregiver perspectives of quality of life in dementia: An investigation of the relationship to behavioural and psychological symptoms in dementia. *Dementia and Geriatric Cognitive Disorders, 26*(2), 138–146. https://doi.org/10.1159/000149584

Jackson, D., Roberts, G., Wu, M. L., Ford, R., & Doyle, C. (2016). A systematic review of the effect of telephone, internet or combined support for carers of people living with Alzheimer's, vascular or mixed dementia in the community. *Archives of Geron-

tology and Geriatrics, 66, 218-236. https://doi.org/10.1016/j.archger.2016.06.013

Joling, K. J., van Marwijk, H. W. J., Veldhuijzen, A. E., van der Horst, H. E., Scheltens, P., Smit, F., & van Hout, H. P. J. (2015). The two-year incidence of depression and anxiety disorders in spousal caregivers of persons with dementia: Who is at the greatest risk? *American Journal of Geriatric Psychiatry, 23*(3), 293-303. https://doi.org/10.1016/j.jagp.2014.05.005

Kaddour, L., & Kishita, N. (2020). Anxiety in informal dementia carers: A meta-analysis of prevalence. *Journal of Geriatric Psychiatry and Neurology, 33*(3), 161-172. https://doi.org/10.1177/0891988719868313

Kaluza, G. (2015). *Stressbewältigung: Trainingsmanual zur psychologischen Gesundheitsförderung* [Stress management: Training manual for psychological health promotion] (3rd ed.). Springer.

Kaluza, G. (2011). *Salute! Was die Seele stark macht: Programm zur Förderung psychosozialer Ressourcen* [Salute! What makes the soul strong: Program for the promotion of psychosocial resources]. Klett-Cotta.

Karg, N., Graessel, E., Randzio, O., & Pendergrass, A. (2018). Dementia as a predictor of care-related quality of life in informal caregivers: A cross-sectional study to investigate differences in health-related outcomes between dementia and non-dementia caregivers. *BMC Geriatrics, 18*(189). https://doi.org/10.1186/s12877-018-0885-1

Kasl-Godley, J. (2003). Anticipatory grief and loss: Implications for intervention. In D. W. Coon, D. Gallagher-Thompson, & L. W. Thompson (Eds.), *Innovative interventions to reduce dementia caregiver distress* (pp. 210-219). Springer.

Kiresuk, T. J., & Sherman, R. E. (1968). Goal Attainment Scaling: A general method for evaluating comprehensive community mental health programs. *Community Mental Health Journal, 4*, 443-453. https://doi.org/10.1007/BF01530764

Kneebone, I. I., & Martin, P. R. (2003). Coping and caregivers of people with dementia. *British Journal of Health Psychology, 8*(1), 1-17. https://doi.org/10.1348/135910703762879174

Kobiske, K. R., Bekhet, A. K., Garnier-Villarreal, M., & Frenn, M. (2019). Predeath grief, resourcefulness, and perceived stress among caregivers of partners with young-onset dementia. *Western Journal of Nursing Research, 41*(7), 973-989. https://doi.org/10.1177/0193945918806689

Kurz, A. (1998). Managing the burden of Alzheimer's disease: A partnership between caregiver and physician. *European Journal of Neurology, 5*, 1-8. https://doi.org/10.1111/j.1468-1331.1998.tb00443.x

Kurz, A., & Wilz, G. (2011). Carer burden in dementia: Origins and intervention. *Der Nervenarzt, 82*(3), 336-342. https://doi.org/10.1007/s00115-010-3108-3

Lammers, C. H. (2011). *Emotionsbezogene Psychotherapie: Grundlagen, Strategien und Techniken* [Emotion-based psychotherapy: Foundations, strategies and techniques] (Vol. 2). Schattauer.

Lamura, G., Mnich, E., Wojszel, B., Nilan, M., Krevers, B., Mestheneos, L., & Dohner, H. (2006). The experience of family carers of older people in the use of support services in Europe: Selected findings from the EUROFAMCARE project. *Zeitschrift für Gerontologie und Geriatrie, 39*(6), 429-442. https://doi.org/10.1007/s00391-006-0416-0

Lee, J., Baik, S., Becker, T., & Cheon, J. (2022). Themes describing social isolation in family caregivers of people living with dementia: A scoping review. *Dementia: International Journal of Social Research and Practice, 21*(2), 701-721. https://doi.org/10.1177/14713012211056288

Liew, T. M., Tai, B. C., Yap, P., & Koh, G. C. H. (2019). Contrasting the risk factors of grief and burden in caregivers of persons with dementia: Multivariate analysis. *International Journal of Geriatric Psychiatry, 34*(2), 258-264. https://doi.org/10.1002/gps.5014

Lindemann, E. (1994). The symptomatology and management of acute grief. *American Journal of Psychiatry, 10*(1), 141-148.

Liu, C., Fabius, C. D., Howard, V. J., Haley, W. E., & Roth, D. L. (2021). Change in social engagement among incident caregivers and controls: Findings from the Caregiving Transitions Study. *Journal of Aging and Health, 33*(1-2), 114-124. https://doi.org/10.1177/0898264320961946

Lopez, J., Romero-Moreno, R., Márquez-González, M., & Losada, A. (2012). Spirituality and self-efficacy in dementia family caregiving: Trust in God and in yourself. *International Psychogeriatrics, 24*(12), 1943-1952. https://doi.org/10.1017/S1041610212001287

Losada, A., Marquez-Gonzalez, M., Knight, B. G., Yanguas, J., Sayegh, P., & Romero-Moreno, R. (2010). Psychosocial factors and caregivers' distress: Effects of familism and dysfunctional thoughts. *Aging & Mental Health, 14*(2), 193-202. https://doi.org/10.1080/13607860903167838

Losada, A., Márquez-González, M., & Romero-Moreno, R. (2011). Mechanisms of action of a psychological intervention for dementia caregivers: Effects of behavioral activation and modification of dysfunctional thoughts. *International Journal of Geriatric Psychiatry, 26*(11), 1119-1127. https://doi.org/10.1002/gps.2648

Losada, A., Marquez-Gonzalez, M., Romero-Moreno, R., Mausbach, B. T., Lopez, J., Fernandez-Fernandez, V., & Nogales-Gonzalez, C. (2015). Cognitive-behavioral therapy (CBT) versus acceptance and commitment therapy (ACT) for dementia family caregivers with significant depressive symptoms: Results of a randomized clinical trial. *Journal of Consulting and Clinical Psychology, 83*(4), 760-772. https://doi.org/10.1016/S1878-7649(14)70088-9

Luoma, J., Hayes, S. C., & Walser, R. D. (2008). *Learning ACT: An acceptance & commitment therapy skills-training manual for therapists*. New Harbinger.

Márquez-González, M., Romero-Moreno, R., Cabrera, I., Olmos, R., Pérez-Miguel, A., & Losada, A. (2020). Tailored versus manualized interventions for dementia caregivers: The functional analysis-guided modular intervention. *Psychology and Aging, 35*(1), 41-54. https://doi.org/10.1037/pag0000412

Marwit, S. J., & Meuser, T. M. (2002). Development and initial validation of an inventory to assess grief in caregivers of persons with Alzheimer's disease. *The Gerontologist, 42*(6), 751-765. https://doi.org/10.1093/geront/42.6.751

Mausbach, B. T., Patterson, T. L., Rabinowitz, Y. G., Grant, I., & Schulz, R. (2007). Depression and distress predict time to cardiovascular disease in dementia caregivers. *Health Psychology, 26*(5), 539-544. https://doi.org/10.1037/0278-6133.26.5.539

McLennon, S. M., Habermann, B., & Rice, M. (2011). Finding meaning as a mediator of burden on the health of caregivers of spouses with dementia. *Aging & Mental Health, 15*(4), 522-530. https://doi.org/10.1080/13607863.2010.543656

McNaughton, M. E., Patterson, T. L., Smith, T. L., & Grant, I. (1995). The relationship among stress, depression, locus of control, irrational beliefs, social support, and health in Alzheimer's disease caregivers. *Journal of Nervous and Mental Disease, 183*(2), 78-85.

Meibert, P., Michalak, J., & Heidenreich, T. (2010). Achtsamkeit in kognitiv-behavioralen Therapien [Mindfulness in cognitive-behavioural therapies]. *Psychotherapie in Psychiatrie, Psychotherapeutischer Medizin und Klinischer Psychologie, 15*(1), 98-114.

Meichsner, F., Schinköthe, D., & Wilz, G. (2016). The Caregiver Grief Scale: Development, exploratory and confirmatory factor analysis, and validation. *Clinical Gerontologist, 39*(4), 342-361. https://doi.org/10.1080/07317115.2015.1121947

Meichsner, F., Theurer, C., & Wilz, G. (2019a). Acceptance and treatment effects of an internet-delivered cognitive-behavioral intervention for family caregivers of people with dementia: A randomized-controlled trial. *Journal of Clinical Psychology, 75*(4), 594-613. https://doi.org/10.1002/jclp.22739

Meichsner, F., Töpfer, N. F., Reder, M., Soellner, R., & Wilz, G. (2019b). Telephone-based cognitive behavioral intervention improves dementia caregivers' quality of life. *American Journal of Alzheimer's Disease and Other Dementias, 34*(4), 236-246. https://doi.org/10.1177/1533317518822100

Meichsner, F., & Wilz, G. (2018). Dementia caregivers' coping with pre-death grief: Effects of a CBT-based intervention. *Aging & Mental Health, 22*(2), 218-225. https://doi.org/10.1080/13607863.2016.1247428

Meuser, T. M., & Marwit, S. J. (2001). A comprehensive, stage-sensitive model of grief in dementia caregiving. *The Gerontologist, 41*(5), 658-670. https://doi.org/10.1093/geront/41.5.658

Meuser, T. M., Marwit, S. J., & Sanders, S. (2004). Assessing grief in family caregivers. In K. J. Doka (Ed.), *Living with grief: Alzheimer's disease* (pp. 169-195). Hospice Foundation of America.

Miller, W. R., & Rollnick, S. (2012). *Motivational interviewing: Helping people change* (3rd ed.). Guilford Publications.

Mittelman, M. S., Roth, D. L., Coon, D. W., & Haley, W. E. (2004). Sustained benefit of supportive intervention for depressive symptoms in caregivers of patients with Alzheimer's disease. *American Journal of Psychiatry, 161*(5), 850-856. https://doi.org/10.1176/appi.ajp.161.5.850

Miyamoto, Y., Ito, H., Otsuka, T., & Kurita, H. (2002). Caregiver burden in mobile and non-mobile demented patients: A comparative study. *International Journal of Geriatric Psychiatry, 17*(8), 765-773. https://doi.org/10.1002/gps.694

Mohr, D. C., Ho, J., Duffecy, J., Reifler, D., Sokol, L., Burns, M. N., Jin, L., & Siddique, J. (2012). Effect of telephone-administered vs face-to-face cognitive behavioral therapy on adherence to therapy and depression outcomes among primary care patients: A randomized trial. *JAMA: The Journal of the American Medical Association, 307*(21), 2278-2285. https://doi.org/10.1001/jama.2012.5588

Monin, J. K., & Schulz, R. (2009). Interpersonal effects of suffering in older adult caregiving relationships. *Psychology and Aging, 24*(3), 681-695. https://doi.org/10.1037/a0016355

Moniz-Cook, E., Vernooij-Dassen, M., Woods, R., Verhey, F., Chattat, R., De Vugt, M., Mountain, G., O'Connell, M., Harrison, J., Vasse, E., Droes, R. M., & Orrell, M. for the Interdem Group. (2008). A European consensus on outcome measures for psychosocial intervention research in dementia care. *Aging & Mental Health, 12*(1), 14-29.

Morgan, D. G., Semchuk, K. M., Stewart, N. J., & D'Arcy, C. (2002). Rural families caring for a relative with dementia: Barriers to use of formal services. *Social Science & Medicine, 55*(7), 1129-1142. https://doi.org/10.1016/S0277-9536(01)00255-6

Naleppa, M. J. (1996). Families and the institutionalized elderly: A review. *Journal of Gerontological Social Work, 27*(1-2), 87-111.

Neville, C., Beattie, E., Fielding, E., & MacAndrew, M. (2015). Literature review: Use of respite by carers of people with dementia. *Health & Social Care in the Community, 23*(1), 51-63. https://doi.org/10.1111/hsc.12095

Nogáles-González, C., Romero-Moreno, R., Losada, A., Márquez-González, M., & Zarit, S. H. (2015). Moderating effect of self-efficacy on the relation between behavior problems in persons with dementia and the distress they cause in caregivers. *Aging & Mental Health, 19*(11), 1022-1030. https://doi.org/10.1080/13607863.2014.995593

Noonan, A. E., & Tennstedt, S. L. (1997). Meaning in caregiving and its contribution to caregiver well-being. *The Gerontologist, 37*(6), 785-794. https://doi.org/10.1093/geront/37.6.785

Pearlin, L. I., Mullan, J. T., Semple, S. J., & Skaff, M. M. (1990). Caregiving and the stress process: An overview of concepts and their measures. *The Gerontologist, 30*(5), 583-594. https://doi.org/10.1093/geront/30.5.583

Perren, S., Schmid, R., & Wettstein, A. (2006). Caregivers' adaptation to change: The impact of increasing impairment of persons suffering from dementia on their caregivers' subjective well-being. *Aging & Mental Health, 10*(5), 539-548. https://doi.org/10.1080/13607860600637844

Pilgram, K., & Tschainer, S. (1999). *"Angebunden rund um die Uhr": Probleme pflegender Angehöriger von Demenzkranken und ihre Entlastung durch die Angehörigenberatung e. V. Nürnberg* ["Accessible around the clock": Problems of caring relatives of dementia patients and their relief by the family counselling service Nuremberg] (2nd ed.). Eigenverlag.

Pinquart, M., & Sörensen, S. (2003). Differences between caregivers and noncaregivers in psychological health and physical health: A meta-analysis. *Psychology and Aging, 18*(2), 250-267. https://doi.org/10.1037/0882-7974.18.2.250

Pinquart, M., & Sörensen, S. (2004). Associations of caregiver stressors and uplifts with subjective well-being and depressive mood: A meta-analytic comparison. *Aging & Mental Health, 8*(5), 438-449. https://doi.org/10.1080/13607860410001725036

Radloff, L. S. (1977). The CES-D Scale: A self-report depression scale for research in the general population. *Applied Psychological Measurement, 1*, 385-401. https://doi.org/10.1177/014662167700100306

Reddemann, L. (2020). *Who you were before trauma: The healing power of imagination for trauma survivors*. The Experiment.

Reis, M., & Nahmiash, D. (1995). Validation of the Caregiver Abuse Screen (CASE). *Canadian Journal on Aging/Revue Canadienne Du Vieillissement, 14*(S2), 45-60. https://doi.org/10.1017/S0714980800005584

Reisberg, B., Borenstein, J., & Salob, S. P. (1987). Behavioural symptoms in Alzheimer's disease: Phenomenology and treatment. *Journal of Clinical Psychiatry, 48*(5), 9-15.

Reisberg, B., Ferris, S. H., Deleon, M. J., & Crook, T. (1988). Global Deterioration Scale (GDS). *Psychopharmacology Bulletin, 24*(4), 661-663.

Reisberg, B., Monteiro, I., Torossian, C., Auer, S., Shulman, M. B., Ghimire, S., Boksay, I., BenArous, F. G., Osorio, R., Vengassery, A., Imran, S., Shaker, H., Noor, S., Naqvi, S., Kenowsky, S., &

Xu, J. (2014). The BEHAVE-AD assessment system: A perspective, a commentary on new findings, and a historical review. *Dementia and Geriatric Cognitive Disorders, 38*(1–2), 89–146.

Risch, A., Mund, M., & Wilz, G. (2022). The Caregiver Thoughts Scale: An instrument to assess functional and dysfunctional thoughts about caregiving. *Clinical Gerontologist*, 1–14. https://doi.org/10.1080/07317115.2022.2153775

Roelands, M., Van Oost, P., & Depoorter, A. (2008). Service use in family caregivers of persons with dementia in Belgium: Psychological and social factors. *Health & Social Care in the Community, 16*(1), 42–53. https://doi.org/10.1111/j.1365-2524.2007.00730.x

Rogers, C.R. (1951). *Client-centered therapy*. Mifflin.

Røsvik, J., Michelet, M., Engedal, K., Bieber, A., Broda, A., Gonçalves-Pereira, M., Hopper, L., Irving, K., Jelley, H., Kerpershoek, L., Meyer, G., Marques, M.J., Portolani, E., Sjölund, B.M., Skoldunger, A., Stephan, A., Verhey, F., de Vugt, M., Woods, B., … Machado, A. (2020). Interventions to enhance access to and utilization of formal community care services for home dwelling persons with dementia and their informal carers: A scoping review. *Aging & Mental Health, 24*(2), 200–211.

Rother, D., & Wilz, G. (2010). *Inanspruchnahme professioneller Hilfe bei pflegenden Angehörigen Demenzerkrankter: Veränderung durch ein therapeutisches Gruppenprogramm* [Use of professional help by family caregivers of dementia patients: Change through a therapeutic group program] [Unpublished bachelor's thesis]. Friedrich-Schiller Universität Jena.

Sachse, R. (2006). *Therapeutische Beziehungsgestaltung* [Complementary relationship building]. Hogrefe.

Sanders, S., Marwit, S.J., Meuser, T.M., & Harrington, P. (2007). Caregiver grief in end-stage dementia: Using the Marwit and Meuser Caregiver Grief Inventory for assessment and intervention in social work practice. *Social Work in Health Care, 46*(1), 47–65. https://doi.org/10.1300/J010v46n01_04

Schacke, C., & Zank, S. (1998). Family care of patients with dementia: Differential significance of specific stress dimensions for the well-being of caregivers and the stability of the home nursing situation. *Zeitschrift für Gerontologie und Geriatrie, 31*(5), 355–361. https://doi.org/10.1007/s003910050059

Schinköthe, D., & Wilz, G. (2014). The assessment of treatment integrity in a cognitive behavioral telephone intervention study with dementia caregivers. *Clinical Gerontologist, 37*(3), 211–234. https://doi.org/10.1080/07317115.2014.886653

Schmidt, R. (2005). Geteilte Verantwortung: Angehörigenarbeit in der vollstationären Pflege und Begleitung von Menschen mit Demenz [Shared responsibility: Work with relatives in full inpatient care and support for people with dementia]. In U. Otto & P. Bauer (Eds.), *Mit Netzwerken professionell zusammenarbeiten* [Working professionally within networks] (pp. 575–616). dgvt-Verlag.

Schoenmakers, B., Buntinx, F., & DeLepeleire, J. (2010). Supporting the dementia family caregiver: The effect of home care intervention on general well-being. *Aging & Mental Health, 14*(1), 44–56. https://doi.org/10.1080/13607860902845533

Schulz, R., & Beach, S.R. (1999). Caregiving as a risk factor for mortality: The caregiver health effects study. *JAMA. Journal of the American Medical Association, 282*(23), 2215–2219. https://doi.org/10.1001/jama.282.23.2215

Schulz, R., Boerner, K., Shear, K., Zhang, S., & Gitlin, L.N. (2006). Predictors of complicated grief among dementia caregivers: A prospective study of bereavement. *American Journal of Geriatric Psychiatry, 14*(8), 650–658. https://doi.org/10.1097/01.JGP.0000203178.44894.db

Schulz, R., Burgio, L., Burns, R., Eisdorfer, C., Gallagher-Thompson, D., Gitlin, L.N., & Mahoney, D.F. (2003). Resources for Enhancing Alzheimer's Caregiver Health (REACH): Overview, site-specific outcomes, and future directions. *The Gerontologist, 43*(4), 514–520. https://doi.org/10.1093/geront/43.4.514

Schulz, R., & Martire, L.M. (2004). Family caregiving of persons with dementia: Prevalence, health effects, and support strategies. *American Journal of Geriatric Psychiatry, 12*(3), 240–249. https://doi.org/10.1097/00019442-200405000-00002

Schulz, R., Savla, J., Czaja, S.J., & Monin, J. (2017). The role of compassion, suffering, and intrusive thoughts in dementia caregiver depression. *Aging & Mental Health, 21*(9), 997–1004. https://doi.org/10.1080/13607863.2016.1191057

Senelick, R.C. (2016). *Living with stroke: A guide for patients and their families* (5th ed.). Healthsouth Press.

Sittler, M.C., Meichsner, F. & Wilz, G. (2020). Evaluation of the factor structure of a German questionnaire version of the behavioral pathology in Alzheimer's disease scale. *Psychotherapie Psychosomatik Medizinische Psychologie PPmP, 70*(03/04), 145–150. https://doi.org/10.1055/a-1067-4733

Stangier, U., Heidenreich, T., & Peitz, M. (2003). *Soziale Phobien. Ein kognitiv-verhaltenstherapeutisches Behandlungsmanual* [Social phobias: A treatment manual based on cognitive-behavioural therapy]. Beltz.

Stephan, A., Bieber, A., Hopper, L., Joyce, R., Irving, K., Zanetti, O., Portolani, E., Kerpershoek, L., Verhey, F., de Vugt, M., Wolfs, C., Eriksen, S., Røsvik, J., Marques, M.J., Gonçalves-Pereira, M., Sjölund, B.M., Jelley, H., Woods, B., & Meyer, G. (2018). Barriers and facilitators to the access to and use of formal dementia care: Findings of a focus group study with people with dementia, informal carers and health and social care professionals in eight European countries. *BMC Geriatrics, 18*(131).

Tarlow, B.J., Wisniewski, S.R., Belle, S.H., Rubert, M., Ory, M.G., & Gallagher-Thompson, D. (2004). Positive aspects of caregiving: Contributions of the REACH project to the development of new measures for Alzheimer's caregiving. *Research on Aging, 26*(4), 429–453. https://doi.org/10.1177/0164027504264493

Theurer, C., & Wilz, G. (2022). Opportunities for fostering a positive therapeutic relationship in an Internet-based cognitive behavioural therapy for dementia caregivers. *Counselling and Psychotherapy Research*. https://doi.org/10.1002/capr.12597

The WHOQOL Group. (1998). Development of the World Health Organization WHOQOL-BREF quality of life assessment. *Psychological Medicine, 28*(3), 551–558. https://doi.org/10.1017/S0033291798006667

Töpfer, N.F., Sittler, M.C., Lechner-Meichsner, F., Theurer, C., & Wilz, G. (2021). Long-term effects of telephone-based cognitive-behavioral intervention for family caregivers of people with dementia: Findings at 3-year follow-up. *Journal of Consulting and Clinical Psychology, 89*(4), 341–349. https://doi.org/10.1037/ccp0000640

Töpfer, N.F., & Wilz, G. (2018). Tele.TAnDem increases the psychosocial resource utilization of dementia caregivers. *GeroPsych: The Journal of Gerontopsychology and Geriatric Psychiatry, 31*(4), 173–183.

Töpfer, N.F., & Wilz, G. (2021). Increases in utilization of psychosocial resources mediate effects of cognitive-behavioural intervention on dementia caregivers' quality of life. *Journal of Positive Psychology, 16*(3), 356–366. https://doi.org/10.1080/17439760.2020.1716047

Töpfer, N. F., Wrede, N., & Wilz, G. (2022). Pragmatic effectiveness of face-to-face Cognitive-Behavioral Therapy for family caregivers of people with dementia. *Clinical Gerontologist.* https://doi.org/10.1080/07317115.2022.2156828

Töpfer, N. F., Wrede, N., Theurer, C., & Wilz, G. (2023). Face-to-face versus telephone-based cognitive-behavioral therapy for family caregivers of people with dementia. *Journal of Clinical Psychology.* https://doi.org/10.1002/jclp.23538

Välimäki, T., Vehviläinen-Julkunen, K., Pietilä, A. M., & Koivisto, A. (2012). Life orientation in Finnish family caregivers' of persons with Alzheimer's disease: A diary study. *Nursing & Health Sciences, 14*(4), 480–487. https://doi.org/10.1111/j.1442-2018.2012.00721.x

van der Linde, R. M., Dening, T., Matthews, F. E., & Brayne, C. (2014). Grouping of behavioural and psychological symptoms of dementia. *International Journal of Geriatric Psychiatry, 29*(6), 562–568. https://doi.org/10.1002/gps.4037

Vandepitte, S., Van Den Noortgate, N., Putman, K., Verhaeghe, S., Verdonck, C., & Annemans, L. (2016). Effectiveness of respite care in supporting informal caregivers of persons with dementia: A systematic review. *International Journal of Geriatric Psychiatry, 31*(12), 1277–1288. https://doi.org/10.1002/gps.4504

Vernooij-Dassen, M., Draskovic, I., McCleery, J., & Downs, M. (2011). Cognitive reframing for carers of people with dementia. *Cochrane Database of Systematic Reviews, 11*, Article CD005318. https://doi.org/10.1002/14651858.CD005318.pub2

Vernooij-Dassen, M. J., Felling, A. J., Brummelkamp, E., Dauzenberg, M. G., van den Bos, G. A., & Grol, R. (1999). Assessment of caregiver's competence in dealing with the burden of caregiving for a dementia patient: A Short Sense of Competence Questionnaire (SSCQ) suitable for clinical practice. *Journal of the American Geriatrics Society, 47*(2), 256–257. https://doi.org/10.1111/j.1532-5415.1999.tb04588.x

Verreault, P., Turcotte, V., Ouellet, M. C., Robichaud, L. A., & Hudon, C. (2021). Efficacy of cognitive-behavioural therapy interventions on reducing burden for caregivers of older adults with a neurocognitive disorder: A systematic review and meta-analysis. *Cognitive Behaviour Therapy, 50*(1), 19–46. https://doi.org/10.1080/16506073.2020.1819867

von Känel, R., Mausbach, B. T., Patterson, T. L., Dimsdale, J. E., Aschbacher, K., Mills, P. J., Ziegler, M. G., Ancoli-Israel, S., & Grant, I. (2008). Increased Framingham coronary heart disease risk score in dementia caregivers relative to non-caregiving controls. *Gerontology, 54*(3), 131–137. https://doi.org/10.1159/000113649

Walker, R. J., Pomeroy, E. C., McNeil, J. S., & Franklin, C. (1995). Anticipatory grief and Alzheimer's disease: Strategies for intervention. *Journal of Gerontological Social Work, 22*(3–4), 21–40. https://doi.org/10.1300/J083V22N03_03

Waller, A., Dilworth, S., Mansfield, E., & Sanson-Fisher, R. (2017). Computer and telephone delivered interventions to support caregivers of people with dementia: A systematic review of research output and quality. *BMC Geriatrics, 17*(265). https://doi.org/10.1186/s12877-017-0654-6

Ware, J. E., & Sherbourne, C. D. (1992). The MOS 36-Item Short-Form Health Survey (SF-36): Conceptual framework and item selection. *Medical Care, 30*(6), 473–483. https://doi.org/10.1097/00005650-199206000-00002

Wasilewski, M. B., Stinson, J. N., & Cameron, J. I. (2017). Web-based health interventions for family caregivers of elderly individuals: A scoping review. *International Journal of Medical Informatics, 103*(Suppl. C), 109–138. https://doi.org/10.1016/j.ijmedinf.2017.04.009

Wawrziczny, E., Pasquier, F., Ducharme, F., Kergoat, M. J., & Antoine, P. (2017). Do spouse caregivers of young and older persons with dementia have different needs? A comparative study. *Psychogeriatrics, 17*(5), 282–291. https://doi.org/10.1111/psyg.12234

Williamson, G. M., & Shaffer, D. R. (2000). Caregiver loss and quality of care provided: Pre-illness relationship makes a difference. In J. H. Harvey & E. D. Miller (Eds.), *Loss and trauma: General and close relationship perspectives* (pp. 307–330). Brunner/Mazel.

Wilz, G., Adler, C., & Gunzelmann, T. (2001). *Gruppenarbeit mit Angehörigen von Demenzkranken. Ein therapeutischer Leitfaden* [Group work with relatives of dementia patients: A therapeutic guide]. Hogrefe.

Wilz, G., Meichsner, F., & Soellner, R. (2017). Are psychotherapeutic effects on family caregivers of people with dementia sustainable? Two-year long-term effects of a telephone-based cognitive behavioral intervention. *Aging & Mental Health, 21*(7), 774–781. https://doi.org/10.1080/13607863.2016.1156646

Wilz, G., Reder, M., Meichsner, F., & Soellner, R. (2018a). The Tele.TAnDem intervention: Telephone-based CBT for family caregivers of people with dementia. *The Gerontologist, 58*(2), 118–129. https://doi.org/10.1093/geront/gnx183

Wilz, G., Schinköthe, D., & Kalytta, T. (2015). *Therapeutische Unterstützung für pflegende Angehörige von Menschen mit Demenz. Das Tele.TAnDem-Behandlungsprogramm* [Teletherapy for family caregivers of people with dementia: The Tele.TAnDem manual]. Hogrefe.

Wilz, G., Schinköthe, D., & Soellner, R. (2011). Goal attainment and treatment compliance in a cognitive-behavioral telephone intervention for family caregivers of persons with dementia. *GeroPsych: The Journal of Gerontopsychology and Geriatric Psychiatry, 24*(3), 115–125. https://doi.org/10.1024/1662-9647/a000043

Wilz, G., & Soellner, R. (2016). Evaluation of a short-term telephone-based cognitive behavioral intervention for dementia family caregivers. *Clinical Gerontologist, 39*(1), 25–47. https://doi.org/10.1080/07317115.2015.1101631

Wilz, G., Weise, L., Reiter, C., Reder, M., Machmer, A., & Soellner, R. (2018b). Intervention helps family caregivers of people with dementia attain own therapy goals. *American Journal of Alzheimer's Disease and Other Dementias, 33*(5), 301–308. https://doi.org/10.1177/1533317518769475

Wimo, A., Gauthier, S., & Prince, M. (2018). *Global estimates of informal care: World Alzheimer report*. Alzheimer's Disease International (ADI) and Karolinska Institute.

Winslow, B. W. (2003). Family caregivers' experiences with community services: A qualitative analysis. *Public Health Nursing, 20*(5), 341–348. https://doi.org/10.1046/j.1525-1446.2003.20502.x

Wittchen, H.-U., & Hoyer, J. (2006). *Klinische Psychologie & Psychotherapie* [Clinical psychology & psychotherapy]. Springer.

Worden, J. W. (2018). *Grief counseling and grief therapy: A handbook for the mental health practitioner* (5th ed.). Springer. https://doi.org/10.1891/9780826134752

Wrede, N., Töpfer, N. F., & Wilz, G. (2023). Effects of general change mechanisms on outcome in telephone-based cognitive-behavioral therapy for distressed family caregivers. *Journal of Clinical Psychology.* https://doi.org/10.1002/jclp.23535

Wu, Q., Yamaguchi, Y., & Greiner, C. (2022). Factors associated with the well-being of family caregivers of people with dementia. *Psychogeriatrics, 22*(2), 218–226. https://doi.org/10.1111/psyg.12805

Xu, L., Liu, Y. W., He, H., Fields, N. L., Ivey, D. L., & Kan, C. (2021). Caregiving intensity and caregiver burden among caregivers of people with dementia: The moderating roles of social support. *Archives of Gerontology and Geriatrics, 94,* Article 104334. https://doi.org/10.1016/j.archger.2020.104334

Zarit, S. H., Femia, E. E., Kim, K., & Whitlatch, C. J. (2010). The structure of risk factors and outcomes for family caregivers: Implications for assessment and treatment. *Aging & Mental Health, 14*(2), 220–231. https://doi.org/10.1080/13607860903167861

Zarit, S. H., Reever, K. E., & Bachpeterson, J. (1980). Relatives of the impaired elderly: Correlates of feelings of burden. *The Gerontologist, 20*(6), 649–655. https://doi.org/10.1093/geront/20.6.649

Zigmond, A. S., & Snaith, R. P. (1983). The Hospital Anxiety and Depression Scale. *Acta Psychiatrica Scandinavica, 67*(6), 361–370. https://doi.org/10.1111/j.1600-0447.1983.tb09716.x

Appendix

The following materials for your book can be downloaded free of charge once you register on the Hogrefe website:

Worksheet 7-1: What Would You Like to Achieve?
Worksheet 7-2: Checklist for Defining a Target State
Worksheet 8-1: ABC Model
Worksheet 9-1: General Tips for Dealing With Difficult Behaviors
Worksheet 9-2: Wandering Around Aimlessly
Worksheet 9-3: Restlessness, Sleep–Wake–Rhythm Disorders
Worksheet 9-4: Constant Questions, Repeating Oneself
Worksheet 9-5: Anxiety
Worksheet 9-6: Accusations, Distrust
Worksheet 9-7: Unfavorable Habits I: Throwing Important Things Away
Worksheet 9-8: Unfavorable Habits II: Searching, Rummaging, Collecting, Hoarding
Worksheet 9-9: Incontinence
Worksheet 9-10: Personal Hygiene
Worksheet 9-11: Feelings of Disgust
Worksheet 9-12: Eating and Drinking
Worksheet 9-13: Problems With Visits to the Doctor
Worksheet 9-14: Driving
Worksheet 9-15: Safety Precautions
Worksheet 9-16: Behavior Analysis
Worksheet 9-17: Behavior Experiment Protocol
Worksheet 10-1: Short Exercise for Coping With Acute Stress
Worksheet 11-1: Scale Model
Worksheet 11-2: Suggestions for Pleasant Activities
Worksheet 11-3: Suggestions for Self-Care
Worksheet 11-4: My Current Weekly Plan
Worksheet 11-5: My New Weekly Plan
Worksheet 11-6: Six Steps for Problem Solving
Worksheet 12-1: List of Our Feelings
Worksheet 13-1: Should I Utilize Support?
Worksheet 13-2: Emergency Plan
Worksheet 13-3: Which Support Is Suitable for My Situation?
Worksheet 14-1: What Should Be Considered When Choosing a Nursing Home?

How to proceed:

1. Go to www.hgf.io/media and create a user account. If you already have one, please log in.
2. Go to **My supplementary materials** in your account dashboard and enter the code below. You will automatically be redirected to the download area, where you can access and download the supplementary materials.

Code: **B-XKD3QM**

To make sure you have permanent direct access to all the materials, we recommend that you download them and save them on your device.

Worksheet 7-1

What Would I Like to Achieve?

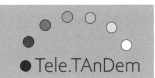

1. Which specific problem should be changed?

2. Which goal should be reached? (Is it attainable in about ___ months?)

3. What do I want to do specifically?

4. How, where, and when do I want to implement it?

5. Who could support me, if necessary?

Worksheet 7-2
Checklist for Defining a Target State

Participant-ID: _____   Name of therapist: _____   Goal-No.: _____

Date when the GAS goal was fully defined: _____   Session No.: _____

1. Selecting the goal
Which specific problem should be changed? _____

2. Formulating the goal
Which goal should be achieved (appropriate and relevant for family caregivers, reachable in _____ months)? _____

3. Goal criteria (only applies to behavior-related goals) – How can one recognize and check the goal attainment (measurable or observable criteria)?

What do you want to do specifically? _____

How, i.e., in what form, do you want to implement it? _____

When/how often do you want to implement it? _____

Where should it occur? _____

Goal Attainment Scale (GAS)

Appraisal	Worsening	Initial state Baseline	Slight improvement	Attainment of the desired target state	Extreme improvement
Caregiver	–1	0	+1	+2	+3
Therapist	–1	0	+1	+2	+3
	• Partial or complete worsening of the defined criteria of the target state	• Stabilization of the initial state • Worsening could be stopped!	• Positive change of the initial state • Partial attainment of the desired goal criteria	• Complete attainment of all desired goal criteria	• Partial or complete attainment of goal, much greater than expected

This page may be reproduced by the purchaser for personal/clinical use. See p. 159 for instructions on how to obtain the printable PDF.
From: G. Wilz: Psychotherapeutic Support for Family Caregivers of People With Dementia: The Tele.TAnDem Manual
© 2024 Hogrefe Publishing

Worksheet 8-1, page 1 of 2

ABC Model

●Tele.TAnDem

Activating event

Briefly describe the situation.

Your belief, your thoughts – your inner self-talk

Recall what you were thinking in the situation. What was on your mind? Which expectations or beliefs did you have?

Consequences and feelings

How did you feel during and afterward or as a result of your inner self-talk – your thoughts? What did you do (or avoid) due to your feelings? What physical reactions can you remember?

(based on Ellis, 1977)

Worksheet 8-1, page 2 of 2

ABC Model

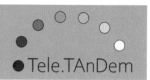

 Activating event

Briefly describe the situation.

I'm away for 2 hours and thinking: Maybe he's not doing well when I'm not there.

 Your belief, your thoughts – your inner self-talk

Recall what you were thinking in the situation. What was on your mind? Which expectations or beliefs did you have?

Then I have a guilty conscience and think: You can't just leave him alone for so long. I'm sure he's not doing well. Hopefully, nothing will happen to him. I often get worried and think: You shouldn't have left him alone.

 Consequences and feelings

How did you feel during and afterward or as a result of your inner self-talk – your thoughts? What did you do (or avoid) due to your feelings? What physical reactions can you remember?

Then I get anxious, feel bad, and can no longer enjoy my time alone, and I do everything very quickly so that I can get back home soon. I am tense and anxious. At home, I'm exhausted and frustrated and also a little angry when he's sitting comfortably in the armchair, and I was in such a hurry.

(based on Ellis, 1977)

Worksheet 9-1

General Tips for Dealing With Difficult Behaviors

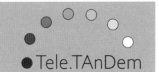

Try to understand the person with dementia and observe their behavior from a "bird's-eye view":
- "Why are they this way today?"
- "What could have triggered it?"

Think about which possibilities to change it exist:
- "Can I change the situation?"
- "Can I change my behavior?"

General strategies:
- Find out more and exchange information with others regarding difficult behaviors, e.g., at information centers, family self-help groups, or on the internet.
- Make sure you provide yourself with balance and relief.
- Make use of support offers.
- Allow yourself time to rest.
- Deal with the disease openly, e.g., in your circle of friends and your neighborhood.
- Talk to the doctors treating your family member.
- Do not confront your family member about their deficits.
- If possible, avoid scolding, criticism, reproach, and pressure to perform.
- Use available resources.
- Make use of helpful aids, such as memory aids (sticky notes).
- Adapt the environment to the changes.

(translated and modified from Deutsche Alzheimer Gesellschaft e.V. Selbsthilfe Demenz
(German Alzheimer Society, self-help dementia), 2012b)

Worksheet 9-2

Wandering Around Aimlessly

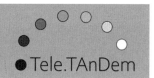

Where is the problem?

"My family member suffering from dementia wants to go away or walks around the apartment anxiously. I constantly have to keep an eye on him."

What may be behind it?

Different causes are possible:
- restlessness, tension, boredom;
- memory disorders and orientation problems regarding time and place, leading to getting lost or wandering around; or
- desire for security, tranquility, and familiar surroundings. Going "home": They no longer recognize their home and want to go to a home from the past.

What can I do?
- Providing explanations usually doesn't help much.
- Set up a comfortable home for your family member with dementia with many memories ("emotional memory"), e.g., by placing photos or objects around the home.
- Keep the person with dementia occupied, e.g., with chores such as folding laundry, drinking coffee together, or looking at photos, reading or sorting the newspaper, singing or playing songs from their childhood.
- Involve the person with dementia in their daily routine.
- Take into account their urge to move and accompany the person with dementia if they want to leave the house.
- Attach a curtain to the front door so it's not recognized as an exit.
- Store shoes, hat, jacket, walker, walking stick, etc., out of sight.
- Attach a bell to the front door so that you can hear if someone leaves.

Further measures:
- Make sure that their name, address, and telephone number are carried with them in case they get lost (e.g., by using a fabric pen, sewing it into the clothing, or by using arm bands, SOS tags, small cards).
- Inform neighbors and acquaintances that they could run away.
- Use technical aids: If necessary, place a mobile phone in their bag or use a person tracking system.
- Have recent photos ready, should a search be necessary.
- Address the person with dementia in a friendly manner from the front, do not touch them or call for them from behind.

(translated and modified from Deutsche Alzheimer Gesellschaft e.V. Selbsthilfe Demenz (German Alzheimer Society, self-help dementia), 2012b)

This page may be reproduced by the purchaser for personal/clinical use. See p. 159 for instructions on how to obtain the printable PDF.
From: G. Wilz: Psychotherapeutic Support for Family Caregivers of People With Dementia: The Tele.TAnDem Manual
© 2024 Hogrefe Publishing

Worksheet 9-3

Restlessness, Sleep–Wake–Rhythm Disorders

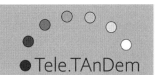

Where is the problem?

"My family member with dementia tends to wander around restlessly at night."

What may be behind it?
Change in the day–night rhythm, e.g., due to:
- disturbances in temporal orientation;
- unfavorable evening bedtime (e.g., already at 6:00 p.m.);
- sleeping a lot throughout the day;
- frequent visits to the toilet at night due to incontinence;
- medication side effects; or
- changes in sleep patterns in old age.

What can I do?
- Ask yourself: Is the wandering around really a problem? Will someone be disturbed? Do they need to be supervised?
- Ensure a normal sleep–wake–rhythm:
  - structured daily routine with activities;
  - daytime exercise and fresh air (walks, dancing);
  - prevent naps and dozing off during the day; and
  - routine bedtime.
- Often tell the person with dementia what time of day it is.
- Everything should be bright during the day and dark at nighttime (but provide orientation light at night to prevent falls).
- Put clothes out of sight at night, and do not let them walk around in pajamas or nightgowns during the day (clearly define what is worn during the day and at night).
- Try sleep rituals: nightcap (tea, hot cocoa), relaxing bath, music, reading (to them).
- If necessary, change the sleeping situation, e.g., separate bedrooms.
- Secure the environment (kitchen, doors, windows).
- Sleep problems and nighttime restlessness may be due to an illness (e.g., acute cold); after the illness improves, the sleep problems improve also.

For sundowning (pronounced restlessness in the late afternoon or the evening):
- Play soothing music before the critical time comes.
- Calm them down with gentle touching for 20–30 minutes beforehand.
- Give them soft pillows, plush animals, or the like for calming down.
- Respond to the restlessness with patience and calmness.
- Caution with sedatives and sleeping pills: Unwanted or paradoxical effects are possible!

(translated and modified from Deutsche Alzheimer Gesellschaft e.V. Selbsthilfe Demenz (German Alzheimer Society, self-help dementia), 2012b)

Worksheet 9-4
Constant Questions, Repeating Oneself

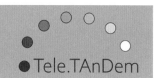

Where is the problem?

"My family member with dementia constantly asks me the same thing!"

What may be behind it?
- Impaired short-term memory; orientation problems regarding place, time, person, and situation; an impaired sense of time; and problems with understanding.

What can I do?
- Do not try using logic or indications such as: "I already told you that 10 minutes ago!" The person with dementia does not remember it.
- Respond to the dementia sufferer's feelings: What's behind it? Perhaps anxiety or insecurity.
- Have patience, stay calm, and provide security and orientation.
- Provide a consistent daily life: Structuring a daily routine and sticking to it helps the person with dementia orient themselves temporally.
- Create orientation aids in the home, e.g., use a symbol or name for each room.
- Inform them about upcoming appointments at short notice to avoid unrest.
- Create rituals.
- Orientation problems on special occasions (such as celebrations, vacations): Create calmness, trust, and orientation (e.g., introduce visitors individually and by name, even if it's their own children; celebrate only in small groups; no longer take vacations abroad but in a familiar environment).

(translated and modified from Deutsche Alzheimer Gesellschaft e.V. Selbsthilfe Demenz
(German Alzheimer Society, self-help dementia), 2012b)

This page may be reproduced by the purchaser for personal/clinical use. See p. 159 for instructions on how to obtain the printable PDF.
From: G. Wilz: Psychotherapeutic Support for Family Caregivers of People With Dementia: The Tele.TAnDem Manual
© 2024 Hogrefe Publishing

Worksheet 9-5

Anxiety

Where is the problem?

"My family member with dementia is afraid (e.g., of getting lost/strangers/new things/being overwhelmed/being alone)."

What may be behind it?
- The person with dementia lives in a world of uncertainty and insecurity. The metaphor "life in a Chinese city" helps to clarify: Imagine that you are suddenly in a foreign county, in a foreign city among people who are unfamiliar to you, whom you do not understand, and whose behavior you cannot classify.
- Orientation and memory problems.
- Misjudgments, hallucinations.
- Insecurity, helplessness.

How can one provide the person with dementia with security and orientation?
- Create a relaxed and familiar atmosphere (familiar pictures, music).
- Provide security and signalize understanding.
- Talk to the person with dementia and convey a sense of security ("I'll be right back!" "All is well." "I'll take care of it, and I'll let you know when everything is in order.")
- Avoid being in a rush and being pressed for time (too many people or appointments).
- Provide security by using scheduled rituals, set times, and structure.
- Create orientation aids: signs, preferably in the form of pictures.
- Involve the person living with dementia, as much as possible in decision-making.
- Use care options (e.g., day care) to ensure continuity and communication opportunities.
- Avoid innovations and environmental changes (change in persons, furniture, technical devices, etc.)
- Avoid changing location.
- If possible, do not leave the person with dementia alone.
- Do not discuss, trivialize, or lecture ("There's nothing there. You're just making that up!"), but react with understanding and trust (e.g., "chasing away" frightening beings together).
- "Where is grandpa?": Gently reveal the "truth" (do not lecture: "Grandpa died years ago. You know that!" For the person with dementia, it may seem like the first time that they are hearing about it due to memory loss.).
- Better: Distract, speak in a friendly manner, and, if necessary, have bodily contact (proximity gives security).

(translated and modified from Deutsche Alzheimer Gesellschaft e.V. Selbsthilfe Demenz
(German Alzheimer Society, self-help dementia), 2012b)

Worksheet 9-6

Accusations, Distrust

Tele.TAnDem

Where is the problem?

"My family member with dementia accuses me of stealing from them and/or throwing away something that belongs to them."

"My family member with dementia accuses me of never visiting them."

"My family member with dementia believes that I just want their money."

What may be behind it?

- Typical accompanying symptoms of dementia:
  - They can no longer remember where they put their things (impaired short-term memory).
  - They have perception disorders and cannot find their things because they does not recognize them (agnosia).
  - They want an explanation for the unusual disappearance, which is troubling them.
  - Self-doubt occurs, and their self-esteem dwindles.
  - Anxiety occurs because the person with dementia experiences their deficits.
  - They want appreciation/recognition (at least not to appear like an "idiot").
  - Because there is no explanation for the person with dementia, someone else must be responsible for the disappearance of the missing things. For the person with dementia, theft is a "logical explanation" for things or money no longer being traceable.
  - Anger, anxiety, accusations, allegations, and distrust result as a consequence.

What can I do?

- Take the behavior seriously, but not personally: Accusations are a symptom of the disease.
- Signalize to the person with dementia that their anger is understandable.
- Think about what the underlying causes could be.
- Do not interrogate or pressure them.
- Do not start discussing or arguing.
- Respond to the person with dementia and put their mind at ease ("We'll think about it together.")
- Help the person with dementia look for and find their missing thing (if the care recipient finds it on their own, their assumption that it was stolen will be confirmed, which leads to distrust).
- Make the person with dementia feel secure by promising them that the object will appear.
- Sometimes distractions help (doing something else).

How can one be preventative?

- Reduce the number of possible hiding places.
- Get a general overview of favorite hiding places (hiding places are "safe places" for the person with dementia: refrigerator, mattress, linen closet).
- Take precautions in dealing with money, e.g., have only small amounts of cash in their wallet or at home.

(translated and modified from Deutsche Alzheimer Gesellschaft e.V. Selbsthilfe Demenz (German Alzheimer Society, self-help dementia), 2012b)

Worksheet 9-7

Unfavorable Habits I: Throwing Important Things Away

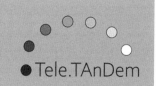

Where is the problem?

"My family member with dementia suddenly takes his dentures out and throws them away."

"The hearing aid constantly disappears. This is already the third one now."

What may be behind it?
- The device/technical aid does not fit properly, causes pain, or is damaged.
- The person with dementia can no longer verbally express the problem with the device/aid and react to it by removing the "annoying device."

What can I do?
- Consult a physician/the specialty shop, inform yourself about the dementia disease, and check whether the fit or wearing comfort can be improved or the device/technical aid can be exchanged.
- In some cases, it is reasonable for the person with dementia to live without the device/aid (dentures, for example, but then: soften the food, switch to food that is easy to swallow, watch out for difficulty in swallowing).

(translated and modified from Deutsche Alzheimer Gesellschaft e.V. Selbsthilfe Demenz
(German Alzheimer Society, self-help dementia), 2012b)

This page may be reproduced by the purchaser for personal/clinical use. See p. 159 for instructions on how to obtain the printable PDF.
From: G. Wilz: Psychotherapeutic Support for Family Caregivers of People With Dementia: The Tele.TAnDem Manual
© 2024 Hogrefe Publishing

Worksheet 9-8

Unfavorable Habits II:
Searching, Rummaging, Collecting, Hoarding

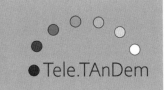

Where is the problem?

"My family member with dementia is constantly looking for something/rummaging around, empties out and puts things back into the cupboards."

"My family member with dementia hoards food for bad times, buys two or three of everything."

What may be behind it?
- Impaired short-term memory: The person with dementia cannot remember where something was put.
- It is difficult for them to keep an overview and to remember, for example, what they have already bought.
- Often, they can no longer distinguish what belongs to whom ("I can still recognize my own cardigan!").
- Collecting might be experienced as something nice and important.

What can I do?
- Make copies of important documents, identification cards, etc., and keep them in a safe place.
- Put the collected things back where they belong.
- Inconspicuously get rid of hoarded, perishable foods.
- Reduce the number of possible hiding places.
- Inspect trash cans etc., before emptying them.
- Purchase more than one of certain things (e.g., eyeglasses, spare keys).

(translated and modified from Deutsche Alzheimer Gesellschaft e.V. Selbsthilfe Demenz
(German Alzheimer Society, self-help dementia), 2012b)

Worksheet 9-9, page 1 of 2

Incontinence

Where is the problem?

"My family member with dementia has urine and stool incontinence. He can no longer manage to make it to the toilet in time. He often misses the toilet. It smells bad in the apartment."

What may be behind it?
- Memory and orientation problems: The person with dementia forgets to go to the toilet on time or does not find the bathroom.
- They can no longer perform the necessary actions: undressing and dressing, positioning incontinence materials correctly, or flushing the toilet.
- There is an infection, physical, or psychological problems that the person with dementia can no longer communicate.
- The person with dementia forgets how to control the sphincter muscles of the bladder and bowel.
- The person with dementia can no longer smell or see well.
- Personal hygiene decreases due to the illness.

What can I do?
- At the first sign, medical evaluation as to whether there are any organic disorders (prostate, prolapse of the uterus, bladder infection).
- Pay attention to the person with dementia's feelings of shame.

At the beginning of incontinence:
- The way to the toilet should be easy to find, not too long, and well lit (especially at night).
- Label toilet doors: legibly, with pictures.
- The person with dementia should wear clothes that are easy to undress (pants with elastic bands, hook-and-loop fasteners).
- Give regular times to use the toilet: after getting up, after meals, before going to bed, and before leaving the house.
- Regularly remind them to use the toilet and take them there (if possible, every 2 hours).
- Pay attention to hints: sitting restlessly, legs wiggling. Then discreetly remind the person with dementia to use the toilet and lead them to it.
- Leave the door to the bathroom open at night and switch on the night light, so that the person with dementia can see what they are looking for.

(translated and modified from Deutsche Alzheimer Gesellschaft e.V. Selbsthilfe Demenz
(German Alzheimer Society, self-help dementia), 2012b)

This page may be reproduced by the purchaser for personal/clinical use. See p. 159 for instructions on how to obtain the printable PDF.
From: G. Wilz: Psychotherapeutic Support for Family Caregivers of People With Dementia: The Tele.TAnDem Manual
© 2024 Hogrefe Publishing

Worksheet 9-9, page 2 of 2

Incontinence

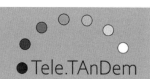

Common problems with incontinence:
- Use of incontinence aids (pads, diapers, diaper pants with or without adhesive closures) that a doctor can prescribe.
- Use of bed pads.
- Important: Talk to the doctor about it!
- Get advice on incontinence aids at the pharmacy. There are also samples to test (size; how does the person in concern cope with it?)
- In case of limited mobility, buy a toilet chair to use at night.

How can you acquaint the person with dementia with incontinence aids?
- Be empathetic, do not hurt/humiliate the dementia sufferer.
- Avoid words like "diaper." It's better to use "disposable briefs" or similar.
- Keep reminding them to go to the toilet despite incontinence aids.
- The person with dementia should be able to dispose of the incontinence aids (e.g., large trash bins in the bathroom).

(translated and modified from Deutsche Alzheimer Gesellschaft e.V. Selbsthilfe Demenz
(German Alzheimer Society, self-help dementia), 2012b)

Worksheet 9-10, page 1 of 2

Personal Hygiene

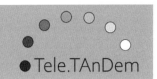

Where is the problem?

"My family member with dementia no longer washes himself regularly. He doesn't shower and gets angry when I want to help him."

What may be behind it?
- Memory problems: They forget personal hygiene in the mornings and later think that they have already taken care of it.
- Impaired perception: Their sense of smell is no longer good, and they, therefore, doesn't notice that their clothes should be changed. They no longer see well and don't notice the stains on their pants.
- They no longer recognize objects or their meaning and handling, e.g., toothbrush, comb, shaving cream.
- Perceiving the loss of independence, of autonomy; feelings of shame.
- Uncomfortable feelings, e.g., due to cold stimuli or water temperature.

What can I do?
- Calmness, patience, and flexibility are important.
- Detach yourself from specific views about personal hygiene (not showering, bathing, or washing oneself daily → drying of the skin due to frequent bathing).
- An occasional sponge bath is justifiable if there are no compelling reasons for a more thorough cleaning (odor, eczema, pressure points).
- Let the person with dementia give themselves the sponge bath under guidance.
- Pay attention to the person with dementia's feelings of shame and mood.
- Adhere to specific circumstances, habits, and rituals (Saturday: bathing day, use favorite soap from the past, pleasant bathroom/water temperature); create consistency.
- Choose a time of day when the resistance is lowest: if possible, in the evening, after dinner, before going to bed.
- Sometimes a bath is more familiar to the person with dementia than a shower.
- Create a relaxed atmosphere, e.g., by singing or playing songs.
- In this relaxed atmosphere, mention that today is bathing day.
- Tell the person with dementia how pleasant a bath can be and that afterward, one not only feels better and fresher but also appears more well-groomed to others.
- Prepare the bath: increase the room temperature, put out anti-slip rugs, and have everything you need ready beforehand (towels, clothing, incontinence aids).
- Explain how to use the tapware and offer help.
- Do not let the water rain down unexpectedly on the person affected (it scares them): better, announce and show each step.

(translated and modified from Deutsche Alzheimer Gesellschaft e.V. Selbsthilfe Demenz
(German Alzheimer Society, self-help dementia), 2012b)

This page may be reproduced by the purchaser for personal/clinical use. See p. 159 for instructions on how to obtain the printable PDF.
From: G. Wilz: Psychotherapeutic Support for Family Caregivers of People With Dementia: The Tele.TAnDem Manual
© 2024 Hogrefe Publishing

Worksheet 9-10, page 2 of 2

Personal Hygiene

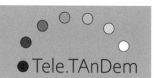

- Ask now and then if everything is okay or keep them company while they are bathing.
- If necessary, offer help: place a washcloth and soap in their hand and lead it to the body/head. If necessary, demonstrate how to do it.
- Dry them off carefully and well, pay attention to pressure sores.
- If necessary, apply lotion or massage their back after the bath.
- Use specific creams and care aids (e.g., disposable washcloths, cleaning sprays – ask your pharmacy about care aids).
- Ensure teeth are brushed, as poor oral hygiene can lead to food intake problems.
- Use external help, and sometimes it is better with outpatient nurses.
- If necessary, use the bathing options in a day-care facility.

(translated and modified from Deutsche Alzheimer Gesellschaft e.V. Selbsthilfe Demenz (German Alzheimer Society, self-help dementia), 2012b)

This page may be reproduced by the purchaser for personal/clinical use. See p. 159 for instructions on how to obtain the printable PDF.
From: G. Wilz: Psychotherapeutic Support for Family Caregivers of People With Dementia: The Tele.TAnDem Manual
© 2024 Hogrefe Publishing

Worksheet 9-11

Feelings of Disgust

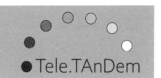

Where is the problem?

"I feel disgusted while eating, and I find incontinence very unpleasant – especially stool incontinence."

What can I do?
- All helpers and caregivers feel similarly, you do not need to be ashamed of that.

→ *In connection with incontinence/personal hygiene:*
- Consistently use disposable gloves made from synthetic material.
- Use aids such as bed pads, specific pillows, cleaning sprays and towels, and disposable washcloths (available at specialty shops for care aids).
- Handle unpleasant tasks as a pair.
- Use external help: It may be that the person with dementia prefers to be helped by a stranger (e.g., clipping toenails, help with washing by an outpatient care service).

→ *In connection with food intake:*
- Detach yourself from previous views regarding eating, e.g., eating with a fork and knife.
- Make sure that the tableware is easy to use (e.g., large handles for gripping the cup) or prepare food that can be eaten with the hands.
- The meals should be easy to chew and swallow.
- Use aids such as eating guards, plates with raised edges, drinking cups, and specific cutlery (available at specialty shops for care aids).
- Eat alone sometimes.

(translated and modified from Deutsche Alzheimer Gesellschaft e.V. Selbsthilfe Demenz
(German Alzheimer Society, self-help dementia), 2012b)

Worksheet 9-12, page 1 of 2

Eating and Drinking

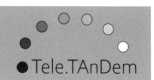

Where is the problem?

"My family member with dementia eats constantly and too much, because they no longer knows that they have already eaten."

"My family member with dementia eats nothing, because they thinks they have already eaten!"

"My family member with dementia no longer knows how to eat with a fork and knife!"

"My family member with dementia does not like the way the food tastes anymore!"

What may be behind it?
- Eating behavior changes.
- Sense of hunger and thirst has changed.
- Changes in the feeling of satiety and taste, e.g., preference only for sweet dishes.
- Memory problems: forgetting what or how much has already been eaten, or forgetting to eat.
- Problems with teeth.
- Physical illnesses.
- Problems with preparation, e.g., unevenly cooked food.
- Problems with handling appliances and utensils, e.g., stove, cutlery.

What can be important for the intake of meals?
- Observe and write down (food and drink: when, what, how much, etc.).
- Check possible causes (e.g., physical illnesses, dental problems).
- Take your time and create a pleasant and calm atmosphere.
- Adhere to regular meal times and create rituals.
- Adapt meals to the needs of the ill person.
- Prepare meals together if possible, e.g., peeling potatoes, setting the table.
- Do not concern yourself with good manners and cleanliness.
- Offer favorite dishes as often as possible.
- Serve individual dishes one after the other to prevent stress in selecting what to eat.
- Perhaps offer foods that are easy to eat with one's fingers.
- Offer heavy, large cutlery so the person with dementia can grasp it better.
- Serve bite-sized food and not too hot.
- Perhaps offer snacks (savory snacks, fruit, vegetables, cookies).
- Keep the person with dementia company while they are eating.
- Provide assistance if necessary: guide their hand (they then may remember the sequence of movements and continue to eat independently).

(translated and modified from Deutsche Alzheimer Gesellschaft e.V. Selbsthilfe Demenz (German Alzheimer Society, self-help dementia), 2012b)

This page may be reproduced by the purchaser for personal/clinical use. See p. 159 for instructions on how to obtain the printable PDF.
From: G. Wilz: Psychotherapeutic Support for Family Caregivers of People With Dementia: The Tele.TAnDem Manual
© 2024 Hogrefe Publishing

Worksheet 9-12, page 2 of 2

Eating and Drinking

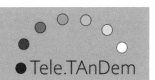

- Remind them to continue eating.
- Well-intentioned instructions such as "chew" or "swallow" may no longer be understood. If so, then show them.
- Provide enough liquids (at least 1.5 liters daily), e.g., colored fruit teas (recognizable as a drink).
- Distribute drinking bottles with glasses throughout the apartment/house (reminder) and always offer it (if necessary, find out what tastes good to the person with dementia).

In case of malnutrition:
- Be certain: check BMI = weight/height2.
- If this is below 21 (>65 years), this indicates malnutrition.
- In this case, encourage appetite and increase nutrient intake.
- Adjust all measures to the needs and habits of the sick person.
- Be considerate of wishes, preferences, and aversions.
- Watch out for changes in taste: Serve both sweet and savory.
- Make food appear appealing (colorful, optically appealing).
- Cozy dining area (clean table and placemats, napkin, clean glass, clean cutlery, good lighting, color contrasts).
- Avoid distractions (radio/TV off).
- Offer high-calorie drinks (malt, cocoa, thickened juices). Thickened juices are also ideal for swallowing difficulties!
- Small bites as snacks between meals.

In case of difficulties in swallowing:
- Visit the doctor or speech therapist for evaluation of swallowing difficulties.
- Use thickened juices (nectars).
- Thicken liquids (remedy for this available at the pharmacy).
- Drink liquids with a straw.
- Use special drinking cups (specialist shop for care aids).
- Purée food or serve liquid or pulpy dishes: creamy soups, egg dishes, spinach, strained vegetables, minced meat dishes, steamed fish filet, mashed potatoes, peas, carrots, pudding, yogurt, milk drinks, boiled fruit, cream cheese, and soft cheeses.
- If necessary, use manufactured baby food (advantage: mild, low acidity, easy to digest).
- Grind medications with a mortar.
- Small portions several times a day.
- Plan enough time to eat.

(translated and modified from Deutsche Alzheimer Gesellschaft e.V. Selbsthilfe Demenz
(German Alzheimer Society, self-help dementia), 2012b)

This page may be reproduced by the purchaser for personal/clinical use. See p. 159 for instructions on how to obtain the printable PDF.
From: G. Wilz: Psychotherapeutic Support for Family Caregivers of People With Dementia: The Tele.TAnDem Manual
© 2024 Hogrefe Publishing

Worksheet 9-13
Problems With Visits to the Doctor

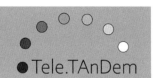

Where is the problem?

"My family member with dementia resists going to the doctor."

"I don't want to see a doctor, because then I will be placed in a home!"

What may be behind it?
- Fear of exposure because the doctor recognizes and identifies deficits.
- Fear of incapacitation, because decisions will be made about one's own person ("I don't want to see a doctor, because then I will be placed in a home!")
- Insecurity: leaving the familiar.
- Uncomfortable examinations.

What can I do?
- Try different ways and possibilities.
- Announce the visit to the doctor several times, not to "bombard" the person with dementia.
- Use simple explanations.
- If there are many worries and fears in advance, announce the visit to the doctor at short notice.
- Plan enough time before the doctor visit so there is no rush.
- Tell the person with dementia that neither the doctor nor you will make any decisions over their head.
- Explain the purpose of the doctor's visit (e.g., to check blood pressure and blood parameters).
- Show that it is a measure of care and responsibility for the loved one: "I am worried about your health, I do not want you to feel bad."
- Stay with them during the doctor's visit and the examinations.
- Explain to the person with dementia in the practice what is happening (applies to the nurses and doctors).
- What is important is the person with dementia's feeling: "They mean well here!"
- Talk to the doctor on the phone in advance.
- Make an appointment with the doctor "together."
- Ask the practice staff for help.
- If necessary, prepare a small note before the doctor's visit, and write down that the patient has dementia and needs special attention and empathy. Give this note to the staff at the reception or the doctor or inform them by telephone in advance. This prevents embarrassing conversations about the behavior and illness in the presence of the person with dementia.
- If possible, organize home visits.

(translated and modified from Deutsche Alzheimer Gesellschaft e.V. Selbsthilfe Demenz
(German Alzheimer Society, self-help dementia), 2012b)

This page may be reproduced by the purchaser for personal/clinical use. See p. 159 for instructions on how to obtain the printable PDF.
From: G. Wilz: Psychotherapeutic Support for Family Caregivers of People With Dementia: The Tele.TAnDem Manual
© 2024 Hogrefe Publishing

Worksheet 9-14
Driving

Where is the problem?

"My family member with dementia refuses to give up driving!"

What may be behind it?
- Symbolizes one's independence and autonomy.
- Lack of the person with dementia's insight into illness: "I don't have anything."
- Limited ability to judge: "I'm still very good at it."

Danger:
- As the disease progresses, road safety decreases.
- Due to the illness, there are limitations in the ability to react, take criticism, and make judgments.
- Concentration, attention, and orientation are impaired.
- Distances can no longer be estimated so well.
- The driver becomes a risk to themselves and others.
- Possibly no insurance coverage in the event of an accident.

What can I do?
- First: Through a conversation, make the person with dementia aware of the dangers.
- Divert the person with dementia from their plan.
- Offer alternatives: "I would like to drive today." "We will walk and take the bus, it's healthier." "We'll take the tram, it's comfortable, and there's no traffic."
- Take the car keys and vehicle registration documents.
- Park the vehicle out of sight so that the person with dementia does not even get the idea of wanting to drive.
- Declare a driving ban by the doctor or have the person with dementia check their fitness to drive (inquire at vehicle inspection agency). A prohibition by a doctor or institution is more likely to be accepted than one by a family member.
- Manipulate something on the vehicle so it no longer starts (e.g., disconnect the battery, unscrew the spark plugs).
- Deregister the vehicle and leave it out of service, sell it because it is "broken," and repairs would be too expensive.
- "Pass" the vehicle on to children and relatives, as they urgently need the car.
- Buy a monthly ticket for the bus, as it is environmentally friendly and cheap.

(translated and modified from Deutsche Alzheimer Gesellschaft e.V. Selbsthilfe Demenz
(German Alzheimer Society, self-help dementia), 2012b)

Worksheet 9-15
Safety Precautions

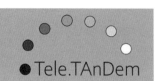

Where is the problem?

"I have to keep my eyes glued to my family member with dementia!"

"He leaves the stove on and goes shopping, eats spoiled food and says that it is still good."

What should I consider?
- Walking and balance disorders, risk of falling.
- Vision and/or hearing problems (check glasses, hearing aid).
- Memory and orientation problems.
- Impaired security awareness and judgment.
- Problem with hazard assessment.
- Misjudgments (e.g., detergent as a drink).
- *Warning:* Danger to oneself and others, risk of fire.

How can I avoid dangerous situations and defuse danger points?
1. Eliminate sources of danger (e.g., stove).
2. Use technical aids (e.g., house emergency call system, stove shutdown).
3. Assess and weigh out dangers and competencies (at regular intervals).

Eliminate sources of danger:
- Remove slippery carpets and rugs.
- Remove sharp edges on cupboards and shelves (there are protective edges for this).
- Remove fragile items (keep glasses, vases, and bowls in a safe place).
- Remove dangerous electrical devices from within reach (kettle, clothing iron, deep fryer, bread slicer, hairdryer, toaster).
- Removing cleaning agents, chemicals, and medication (lock away, possible risk of poisoning).
- Remove inedible food (check the refrigerator regularly).
- Remove lighters and matches (do not leave them lying around).
- Remove keys, especially the car keys.
- No keys on room doors (Danger: Person living with dementia could lock themselves in and will be unable to come out).

Helpful:
- Nonslip mats on stairs.
- Good lighting.
- No slippery floors.
- Make the glass part on glass doors visible.
- Secure stairs, windows, and balconies (danger of falling).
- Attach handles in the bathroom (risk of slipping).
- Nonslip mat in the bath or shower.
- Smoke alarm, smoking under supervision (fire hazard).

(translated and modified from Deutsche Alzheimer Gesellschaft e.V. Selbsthilfe Demenz
(German Alzheimer Society, self-help dementia), 2012b)

Worksheet 9-16

Behavior Analysis

The situation:

My reaction:

My thoughts:

My feelings:

My body:

My behavior:

The consequences:

Worksheet 9-17, page 1 of 2

Behavior Experiment Protocol

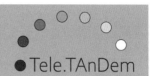

Situation and your task:

Prediction:

What exactly do you expect to happen?

How convinced are you that your expectations will come true (0–10)?

Test the predictions:

What should you pay attention to?

Result:

What actually happened?

Which of your predictions came true, and which did not (in %)?

Conclusion

What did you learn from it?

Have your beliefs changed?

(Protocol sheet translated and modified from Stangier et al., 2003, p. 180)

Worksheet 9-17, page 2 of 2

Behavior Experiment Protocol

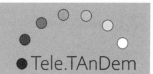

Situation and your task:

Go to a restaurant with your husband (suffering from dementia).

Prediction:

What exactly do you expect to happen?

People will look at us strangely, constantly look over at us and talk about us (put their heads together, whisper)

How convinced are you that your expectations will come true (0–10)?

9

Test the predictions:

What should you pay attention to?

Pay attention to the reactions of the other guests in the restaurant (whether they look over at us, whisper, or look strangely).

Result:

What actually happened?

The other guests were more occupied with themselves. Hardly anyone paid attention to us, not even when my husband got really loud or spilled his drink. Some people took a quick look but went straight back to their food.

Which of your predictions came true, and which did not (in %)?

Other guests look over at us (50%)
Other guests look at us strangely (0%)
Other guests talk about us (0%)

Conclusion

What did you learn from it?

Other guests are busy with themselves, hardly interested, and, if so, they don't find me and my husband strange.

Have your beliefs changed?

I can go out to dinner with my husband and feel good about it.

(Protocol sheet translated and modified from Stangier et al., 2003, p. 180)

This page may be reproduced by the purchaser for personal/clinical use. See p. 159 for instructions on how to obtain the printable PDF.
From: G. Wilz: Psychotherapeutic Support for Family Caregivers of People With Dementia: The Tele.TAnDem Manual
© 2024 Hogrefe Publishing

Worksheet 10-1, page 1 of 2

Short Exercise for Coping With Acute Stress

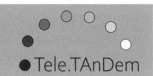

If you end up in a burdensome situation, try to react the following way:

1. **ACCEPT** the burden, e.g., the aggressive behavior of the person with dementia.
   Take the behavior as it is – as part of dementia, as part of your caregiving routine. Anger, accusations, and feelings of guilt help just as little as not wanting it to be true. Accepting the situation includes two things: (1) recognizing signals as early as possible that indicate a difficult situation; and (2) a clear and conscious decision for acceptance (and against fighting with reality).

2. **COOLING DOWN.** Try to get a grip on your own strong agitation when you are "beside yourself," "want to go through the roof," or when you no longer know "if you are on your head or your heels." The point here is to compose yourself, ground yourself, and keep a clear head. How can this be done? By consciously choosing to cool down and against getting worked up about the agitation.
   Cooling down can be reached through targeted, short exercises, e.g., through conscious, prolonged exhaling, with which the "steam" is released. But it can also be a short relaxation or movement exercise.

   My possibilities for cooling down in an acutely burdensome situation:

   _____

   _____

   _____

3. **ANALYZING** the burdensome situation: Take a short moment to come to a conscious and quick assessment of the situation. You can do this by asking yourself: *Can I do/change something at the moment?*

4. **DISTRACTION or ACTION**
   If there is **nothing**, you can do at the moment, distract yourself: take a break, listen to music, think of something pleasant, give someone a call, etc.
   If there is **anything** you can do at the moment, take action: find support, make appointments, etc.

(translated and modified from Kaluza, 2015)

This page may be reproduced by the purchaser for personal/clinical use. See p. 159 for instructions on how to obtain the printable PDF.
From: G. Wilz: Psychotherapeutic Support for Family Caregivers of People With Dementia: The Tele.TAnDem Manual
© 2024 Hogrefe Publishing

Worksheet 10-1, page 2 of 2

Short Exercise for Coping With Acute Stress

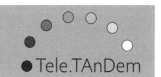

Accept burden

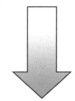

Cool down

Can I change something at the moment?

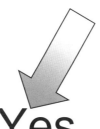 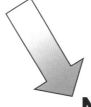

Yes 　　 No

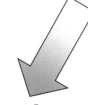 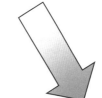

Action 　　 Distraction

(translated and modified from Kaluza, 2015)

Worksheet 11-1

Scale Model

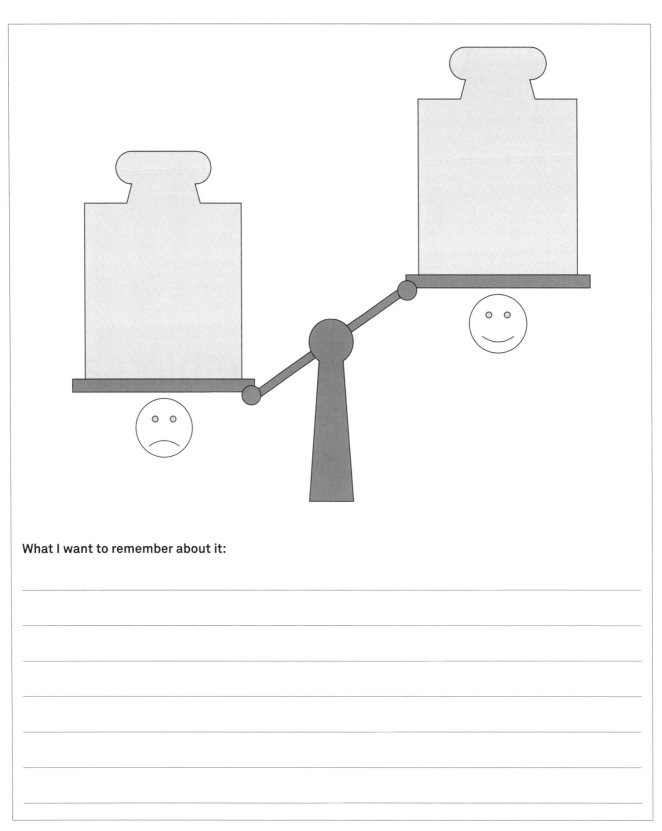

What I want to remember about it:

_____
_____
_____
_____
_____
_____

This page may be reproduced by the purchaser for personal/clinical use. See p. 159 for instructions on how to obtain the printable PDF.
From: G. Wilz: Psychotherapeutic Support for Family Caregivers of People With Dementia: The Tele.TAnDem Manual
© 2024 Hogrefe Publishing

Worksheet 11-2

Suggestions for Pleasant Activities

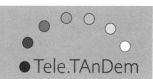

Own ideas …	Pleasant?	
	yes	no
Suggestions …		
Go to the countryside		
Go to a sporting event		
Talk about sports or do sports		
Read tips and advice on self-help		
Make a new acquaintance		
Read novels, short stories, plays, or poems		
Go to lectures/readings		
Plan excursions or vacations		
Listen to music		
Buy something for oneself		
Be artistic (paint, draw, take photos)		
Make someone happy		
Watch TV or listen to the radio		
Clean or rearrange a room or the house		
Talk to yourself		
Have a good conversation		
Work on technical things (cars, bicycles, household appliances, etc.)		
Solve puzzles, crosswords, etc.		
Go eat with friends and acquaintances		
Drink coffee		
Take a shower or a bath		
Take a nap		
Engage with animals, observe animals		
Be with friends		
Just sit around and think		
Make/get yourself something delicious to eat		
Gardening		
Stroll around town		
Visit a museum or exhibition		
Write a diary		
Find silence		
Be alone		
Visit friends		

(translated and modified from Hautzinger, 2000; p. 75 ff.)

This page may be reproduced by the purchaser for personal/clinical use. See p. 159 for instructions on how to obtain the printable PDF.
From: G. Wilz: Psychotherapeutic Support for Family Caregivers of People With Dementia: The Tele.TAnDem Manual
© 2024 Hogrefe Publishing

Worksheet 11-3

Suggestions for Self-Care

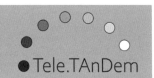

	Important?	
	yes	no
Eat a regular and healthy diet		
Get enough sleep		
Pay attention to the signals from the body		
Get medical checkups		
Exercise, be physically active		
Get a massage		
Sing		
Wear comfortable clothes		
Go on vacation		
Spend time with pleasant people		
Maintain important personal relationships		
Look for opportunities to laugh and enjoy life		
Take time to enjoy		
Say good things to yourself		
Play with children		
Spend time with animals		
Read your favorite books again		
Allow yourself to cry		
Express anger about social grievances through social campaigns, letters, donations, rallies		
Take time to think and empathize		
Write a diary		
Pay attention to your own thoughts, opinions, and feelings		
Open your mind to new areas		
Accept support		
Say "no" to additional responsibilities		
Spend time in nature		
Cultivate optimism and hope		
Be mindful of nonmaterial aspects of life		
Give personal values a place in your own life		
Live out what suits you: meditation, prayer, singing, art		
Contribute in a practical way to things you believe in		
My own ideas:		

This page may be reproduced by the purchaser for personal/clinical use. See p. 159 for instructions on how to obtain the printable PDF.
From: G. Wilz: Psychotherapeutic Support for Family Caregivers of People With Dementia: The Tele.TAnDem Manual
© 2024 Hogrefe Publishing

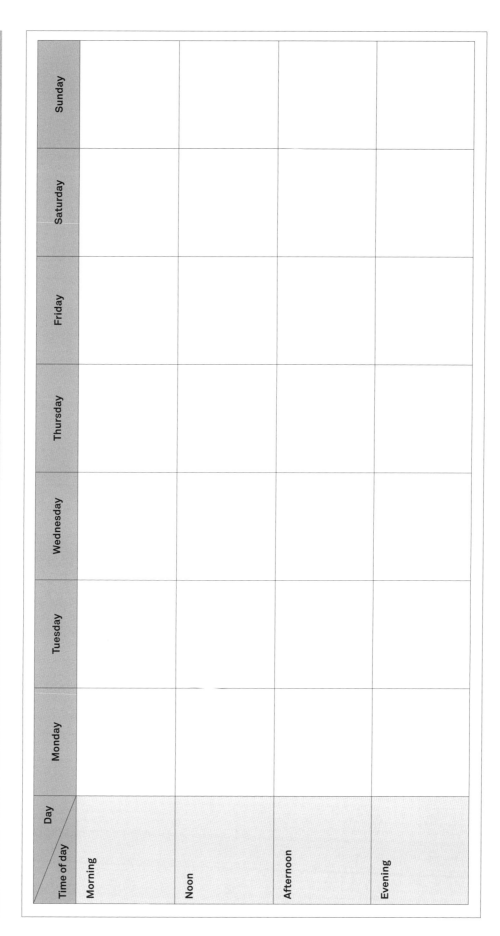

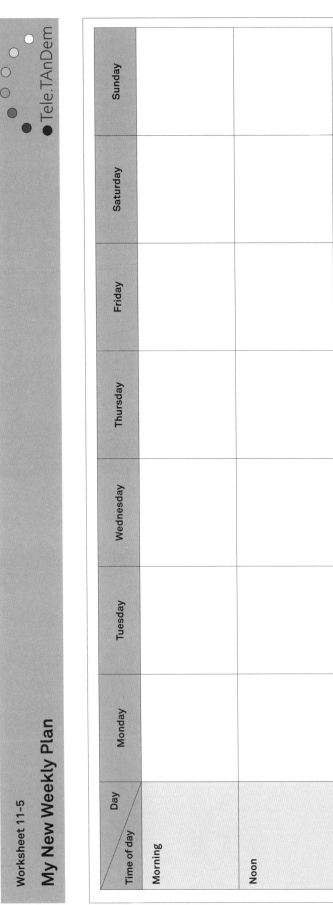

Worksheet 11-6, page 1 of 2

Six Steps for Problem Solving

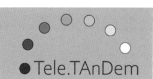

1. What is the problem?
   _____
   _____
   _____
   _____

2. What do I want to achieve?
   _____
   _____
   _____
   _____

3. What solutions are there?
   - _____   - _____
   - _____   - _____
   - _____   - _____
   - _____

4. Consider each suggestion's advantages and disadvantages (next sheet)!

5. Which solution(s) do I find best?
   → _____
   _____

6. How can I implement the best possible solution?

	Task:	Implementation successful?
1st step		
2nd step		
3rd step		
4th step		
5th step		
6th step		

(based on D'Zurilla & Goldfried, 1971)

Worksheet 11-6, page 2 of 2

Six Steps for Problem Solving

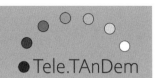

Consider each suggestion's advantages and disadvantages:

Suggestion 1:
Advantages:
_____
_____
_____

Disadvantages:
_____
_____
_____

Suggestion 2:
Advantages:
_____
_____
_____

Disadvantages:
_____
_____
_____

Suggestion 3:
Advantages:
_____
_____
_____

Disadvantages:
_____
_____
_____

Remarks:
_____
_____
_____

(based on D'Zurilla & Goldfried, 1971)

Worksheet 11-6, page 1 of 2

Six Steps for Problem Solving

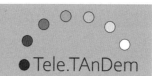

1. What is the problem?

I would like to go on vacation with my husband, but that is impossible because I have no one to care for my mother during the time I'm away.

2. What do I want to achieve?

To go on vacation with my husband twice a year.

3. What solutions are there?

- Place mother in short-term care.
- Ask sister if she will move in for the time.
- Ask a friend if she can check on her every day and have the nursing service come more often.

4. Consider each suggestion's advantages and disadvantages (next sheet)!

5. Which solution(s) do I find best?

→ Place mother in short-term care.

6. How can I implement the best possible solution?

	Task:	Implementation successful?
1st step	Pick out different nursing homes.	Yes
2nd step	Call nursing homes and ask for an appointment.	Yes
3rd step	Visit nursing homes.	Yes
4th step	Decide on the best home and check whether it is available for the desired time.	Yes
5th step	Prepare mother for short-term care.	No
6th step		

(based on D'Zurilla & Goldfried, 1971)

Worksheet 11-6, page 2 of 2

Six Steps for Problem Solving

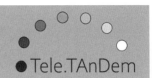

Consider each suggestion's advantages and disadvantages:

Suggestion 1:
Advantages:

Mother would be well looked after. I could enjoy the vacation because I know she would be taken care of.

Disadvantages:

Mother would be in an unfamiliar environment that might break her down even more. She will be scared for the first few days, which makes me feel guilty.

Suggestion 2:
Advantages:

My mother would be in familiar surroundings; my sister would look after her well.

Disadvantages:

My sister would be separated from her family for a week or two. She would have to take a vacation for this time, which makes me feel guilty.

Suggestion 3:
Advantages:

My mother would be in her familiar surroundings; my sister doesn't have to take a vacation. The nursing staff would take good care of my mother. My mother likes my friend; she would get along well with her.

Disadvantages:

My mother would be alone at night, I would have no rest, and I wouldn't be able to enjoy my vacation so well.

Remarks:

_____
_____
_____

(based on D'Zurilla & Goldfried, 1971)

Worksheet 12-1

List of Our Feelings

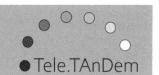

aversion   abhorrence   anger   aggression   amusement   anxiety

condolence   sorrow   gloominess   desire   enthusiasm

merriment   buoyancy   unease   somberness   concern

admiration   gratitude   reverence   jealousy   loneliness   disgust

humiliation   dismay   disappointment   moved   relief

fear   irritability   luck   grouchiness   resentment   hate   homesickness

cheerfulness   boredom   emptiness   passion   love   desire   displeasure

discord   mistrust   empathy   sympathy   envy   curiosity

despondence   panic   helplessness   remorse   affection

gloat   shame   pain   shock   guilt   melancholy

yearning   worry   tension   astonishment   pride   grief   sadness

restlessness   insecurity   contempt   annoyance   admiration   enjoyment

trust   amazement   despair   warmth   wistfulness   distaste

well-being   goodwill   fury   tenderness   rage   satisfaction

fondness   confidence

(translated and modified from Lammers, 2011, p. 337)

Worksheet 13-1

Should I Utilize Support?

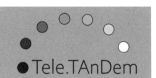

Pros and Cons

	Positive aspects	Negative aspects
If I continue to look after and care for them as before:		
If I utilize support:		

(based on Miller & Rollnick, 2012)

Worksheet 13-2, page 1 of 2

Emergency Plan

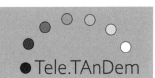

Take the time to plan your procedure in the event of an emergency. Write down who will help you in possible emergencies. Keep the emergency plan in a place that is easy to find in your home.

→ **Remain calm!**

→ **Contact Primary Care Physician/Specialist Physician/Hospital:**

Primary care physician	Address	Telephone
Specialist physician	Address	Telephone
Hospital	Address	Telephone

The hospital emergency department is open around the clock!

→ **…or contact emergency services:**

Police	
Fire department	
Medical on-call service	
Pharmacy emergency service	
Poison control center	
Block ATM and credit cards	

In the event of an emergency, always state:
- Who is reporting the emergency?
- Where did the emergency occur?
- What happened?
- What type of injury occurred (e.g. loss of consciousness, shortness of breath)?
- Wait for further questions!

→ **Contact or inform family/friends:**

Family	Address	Telephone
Friends/Neighbors	Address	Telephone

→ **If necessary, notify a taxi service:**

Taxi	Telephone

Always have a "taxi wallet" ready with the appropriate amount of money needed.

This page may be reproduced by the purchaser for personal/clinical use. See p. 159 for instructions on how to obtain the printable PDF.
From: G. Wilz: Psychotherapeutic Support for Family Caregivers of People With Dementia: The Tele.TAnDem Manual
© 2024 Hogrefe Publishing

Worksheet 13-2, page 2 of 2

Emergency Plan

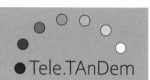

→ **Helpful contact points:**

Local Alzheimer's Society or Association	Telephone _____
	Email _____
	Website _____
Emotional Support Hotline	Telephone _____
	Email _____
	Website _____
Nursing Support	Telephone _____
	Email _____
	Website _____

→ **Personal emergency plan:**

	In case something happens to me:	In case something happens to my family member with dementia:
1st step:		
2nd step:		
3rd step:		
4th step:		
5th step:		
6th step:		

This page may be reproduced by the purchaser for personal/clinical use. See p. 159 for instructions on how to obtain the printable PDF.
From: G. Wilz: Psychotherapeutic Support for Family Caregivers of People With Dementia: The Tele.TAnDem Manual
© 2024 Hogrefe Publishing

Worksheet 13-3

Which Support Is Suitable for My Situation?

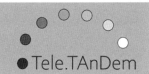

My wish list …

When do I need support? (at what time and in which situations)

Who could support me? What should or could others do for me?

Which costs and limits am I willing to accept?

Worksheet 14-1

What Should Be Considered When Choosing a Nursing Home?

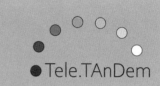

If you want to place a family member living with dementia in a nursing home, you should research nursing homes in your region in a timely manner (sometimes there are waiting lists) and make an appointment with the nursing home. While visiting the home, particular attention should be paid to the following points:

- Does the home have a care concept that considers the special needs and behavior of people living with dementia?
- If family members are involved, will their knowledge on the person living with dementia's behavior and likes and dislikes be used?
- Is there a day structure provided with the care for the residents, or are they left to their own resources?
- Are there offers to bring the residents into action, e.g., through singing, making music, dancing, exercise, going for walks, other activities, spending time with animals?
- What is the atmosphere and tone like in the home? Are the residents treated with dignity and respect?
- What is the size of the rooms and how are they configured? Can residents bring their own furniture? Is there an outdoor area that can be used?
- How are restrictive measures dealt with?
- A sample nursing-home contract with a detailed description of all services and costs should be read carefully before signing the final contract.

What else do I want to know about the nursing home?

_____

_____

_____

(translated and modified from Deutsche Alzheimer Gesellschaft e.V. Selbsthilfe Demenz
(German Alzheimer Society, self-help dementia), 2019)

This page may be reproduced by the purchaser for personal/clinical use. See p. 159 for instructions on how to obtain the printable PDF.
From: G. Wilz: Psychotherapeutic Support for Family Caregivers of People With Dementia: The Tele.TAnDem Manual
© 2024 Hogrefe Publishing

Supporting family caregivers on maintaining positive mental health

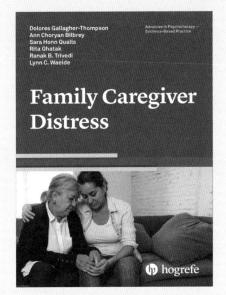

Dolores Gallagher-Thompson / Ann Choryan Bilbrey / Sara Honn Qualls / Rita Ghatak / Ranak B. Trivedi / Lynn C. Waelde

Family Caregiver Distress

This is the first book that takes a "deep dive" to answer the questions that mental health providers encounter when working with family caregivers. Just what are the unique issues family caregivers face? How does this impact their mental health? What can providers do to help?

Based on research and clinical experiences of the authors, this volume in our Advances in Psychotherapy series focuses on examining the specific issues that caregivers of people with Alzheimer's disease or other forms of dementia face. Practitioners learn about the best tools for assessment and which evidence-based interventions help reduce caregiver distress – including cognitive behavioral therapy, acceptance and commitment therapy, and mindfulness and multicomponent intervention programs.

Resources in the appendix include a caretaker intake interview, and the book is interspersed with clinical vignettes that highlight issues of diversity, equity, and inclusion – making this is an essential text for mental health providers from a variety of disciplines including psychology, psychiatry, nursing, social work, marriage and family counseling, as well as trainees in these disciplines.

*Advances in Psychotherapy –
Evidence-Based Practice, vol. 50
2023, xii + 100 pp.,
$29.80 / € 24.95
ISBN 978-0-88937-517-8
Also available as eBook*

"This book synthesizes decades of research and clinical wisdom into brief, actionable steps, and a telling case vignette to convey state-of-the-art assessment and intervention strategies."

Barry J. Jacobs, PsyD, Principal, Health Management Associates, Philadelphia, PA; Co-Author of *AARP Meditations for Caregivers*

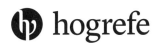

Expert guidance on working psychologically with older adults

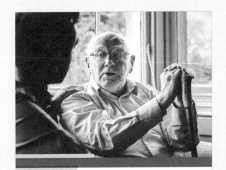

Nancy A. Pachana / Victor Molinari / Larry W. Thompson / Dolores Gallagher-Thompson (Eds.)

Psychological Assessment and Treatment of Older Adults

Mental health practitioners are encountering an ever-growing number of older adults and so an up-to-date and comprehensive text addressing the special considerations that arise in the psychological assessment and treatment of this population is vital.

This accessible handbook does just that by introducing the key topics that psychologists and other health professionals face when working with older adults. Each area is introduced and then the special considerations for older adults are explored, including specific ethical and healthcare system issues. The use of case examples brings the topics further to life. An important feature of the book is the interweaving of diversity issues (culture, race, sexuality, etc.) within the text to lend an inclusive, contemporary insight into these important practice components. The Pikes Peak Geropsychology Knowledge and Skill Assessment Tool is included in an appendix so readers can test their knowledge, which will be helpful for those aiming for board certification in geropsychology (ABGERO).

This is an ideal text for mental health professionals transitioning to work with older clients, for those wanting to improve their knowledge for their regular practice, and for trainees or young clinicians just starting out.

2021, xiv + 266 pp.,
$59.00 / € 50.95
ISBN 978-0-88937-571-0
Also available as eBook

"An important and timely book with a stellar roster of contributors to address key topics regarding mental health practice with older adults. Highly recommended!"

Daniel L. Segal, PhD, Department of Psychology, University of Colorado at Colorado Springs, CO, USA

www.hogrefe.com

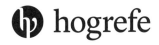

Helping older adults to overcome their unhealthy alcohol use

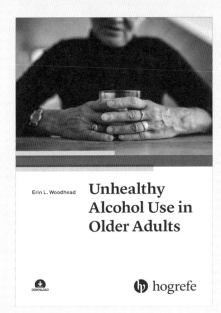

Erin L. Woodhead

Unhealthy Alcohol Use in Older Adults

As our population ages, practitioners find themselves working with older adults more frequently. Alcohol use problems among older adults are often underdiagnosed and undertreated, and there are few treatments designed specifically for this client group. This practical guide provides practitioners with up-to-date information on assessing and treating unhealthy alcohol use among older adults. With a focus on evidence-based treatments, it is highly relevant to practitioners working across a variety of settings. Through the author's expertise, we learn about the prevalence of alcohol use among older adults, the models for understanding unhealthy use, and the different screening and assessment options as well as the treatment possibilities relevant to health care and social service providers. Assessment and treatment options highlight the need to consider lifespan development when providing care as well as the relevance of common life transitions and generational differences. Clinical pearls and vignettes illuminate treatment approaches and further sections discuss pharmacological interventions and cultural considerations. Printable tools are available in an appendix. This book is a must for practitioners from diverse settings who work with older adults.

2024, x + 110 pp.,
$29.80 / € 25.95
ISBN 978-0-88937-510-9
Also available as eBook

The materials for this book can be downloaded from the Hogrefe website after registration.

"This is a must-read for every mental health practitioner who works with older adults. Both experienced clinicians and graduate students entering the field will appreciate this well-written guide as an essential, easy-to-read resource on this increasingly important topic"

Brian Yochim, PhD, ABPP, Board Certified in Clinical Neuropsychology, San Francisco VA Health Care System and University of California, San Francisco (UCSF), CA

www.hogrefe.com

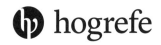